AGING WELL WITH DIABETES

A Johns Hopkins Press Health Book

Aging Well with Diabetes

A 10-POINT ACTION PLAN FOR OLDER ADULTS

Medha Munshi, MD
and
Sheri Colberg, PhD

JOHNS HOPKINS UNIVERSITY PRESS
Baltimore

Note to the Reader: This book is not meant to substitute for medical care and treatment should not be based solely on its contents. Instead, treatment must be developed in a dialogue between the individual and his or her physician. Our book has been written to help with that dialogue.

Drug dosage: The author and publisher have made reasonable efforts to determine that the selection of drugs discussed in this text conform to the practices of the general medical community. The medications described do not necessarily have specific approval by the US Food and Drug Administration for use in the diseases for which they are recommended. In view of ongoing research, changes in governmental regulation, and the constant flow of information relating to drug therapy and drug reactions, the reader is urged to check the package insert of each drug for any change in indications and dosage and for warnings and precautions. This is particularly important when the recommended agent is a new and/or infrequently used drug.

© 2025 Johns Hopkins University Press
All rights reserved. Published 2025
Printed in the United States of America on acid-free paper
9 8 7 6 5 4 3 2 1

Johns Hopkins University Press
2715 North Charles Street
Baltimore, Maryland 21218
www.press.jhu.edu

Library of Congress Cataloging-in-Publication Data is available.

A catalog record for this book is available from the British Library.

ISBN 978-1-4214-5151-0 (hardcover)
ISBN 978-1-4214-5152-7 (paperback)
ISBN 978-1-4214-5153-4 (ebook)

Special discounts are available for bulk purchases of this book. For more information, please contact Special Sales at specialsales@jh.edu.

Contents

Foreword   vii

Introduction	1
Step 1: Change Your Sweetness	12
Step 2: Reverse Your Road to Diabetes	38
Step 3: Stand Up and Stride Away	56
Step 4: Boost Your Gut Health and Your Diet	107
Step 5: Take a Medication Inventory	144
Step 6: Achieve Your Desired Body Weight	172
Step 7: Rev Up Your Brain Power	194
Step 8: Sleep Well, Rest, and Recuperate	215
Step 9: Keep Other Diseases at Bay	231
Step 10: Stay Strong, Stable, and Safe	258

Final Thoughts   281
Notes   285
Appendices and Resources   303
Index   345

Foreword

Aging is a natural journey that each of us embarks upon, filled with its own unique set of experiences, challenges, and joys. For those living with diabetes, this journey can seem particularly daunting. Too often, aging leads to physical limitations and chronic health conditions that can negatively impact quality of life in older adults and limit their ability to take care of themselves. Having diabetes can make other health issues worse, and other health issues can arise after a diabetes diagnosis, but it does not have to be that way. Aging well with diabetes is not only possible, but it can also be a path to discovering deeper resilience, strength, and a renewed zest for life.

Aging Well with Diabetes is dedicated to everyone who is navigating the complexities of aging with diabetes. It aims to provide practical insights, compassionate guidance, and empowering strategies to help you thrive. Living with a chronic condition like diabetes requires vigilant management and self-care, but it also presents an opportunity to cultivate a profound understanding of your own body and health.

Dr. Medha Munshi and Dr. Sheri Colberg explore various aspects of diabetes management, from understanding the intricacies of blood glucose management to the importance of nutrition, exercise, and mental health. *Aging Well with Diabetes* presents an innovative ten-step action plan to help older adults with diabetes—whether they are new to this disease or long-time veterans—to live their best lives possible. It can also assist anyone who cares for older people with diabetes—whether it be family members, friends, neighbors, or health care providers—to better understand how to help these individuals manage their health as well.

VIII • FOREWORD

Aging Well with Diabetes is about more than just managing symptoms; it's about embracing life fully and living with purpose. It's about finding joy in the everyday moments, staying connected with loved ones, and continuing to pursue your passions and dreams. It's about realizing that your condition does not define you but is merely one part of the rich tapestry of your life.

As you read this book, I encourage you to approach it with an open heart and mind. Let it be a source of comfort, encouragement, and inspiration. Remember that you are not alone on this journey— there is a community of individuals and health care professionals ready to support you every step of the way.

May this book serve as a beacon of hope and a practical guide to aging well with diabetes. May it empower you to live a vibrant, fulfilling life, no matter your age or circumstance. Following the ten vital steps in this program will help people live longer with greater vitality and independence with any type of diabetes or associated health issues. Welcome to a new chapter of possibility and well-being.

Osama Hamdy, MD, PhD
Associate Professor of Medicine
Harvard Medical School

AGING WELL WITH DIABETES

INTRODUCTION

If you're reading this, it means you either have a personal interest in aging well—despite having diabetes—or you are a family member, friend, neighbor, caregiver, or health care worker interested in learning as much as possible about growing older with diabetes. In that case, this book is for you.

Almost no one else knows aging and diabetes as well as Dr. Medha Munshi. She is not only a geriatrician (a doctor specializing in older adult care) but also an endocrinologist who focuses primarily on treating patients with diabetes. At the Joslin Diabetes Center affiliated with Harvard University in Cambridge, Massachusetts, she founded a geriatric diabetes clinic to help older adults living with diabetes get the best care possible. This book is the culmination of her years of education, training, and practical experience working with patients—packaged into an innovative 10-step action plan to boost your know-how about living better with diabetes well into your golden years. It's based on the Joslin Geriatric Diabetes Program, so you know it's backed by decades of scientific research and clinical experience that you really can't get anywhere else.

Dr. Sheri Colberg adds her expertise as an exercise physiologist who has conducted numerous studies on diabetes and exercise, aging well, and lifestyle improvements. She has written about these topics extensively, including in a prior book on aging well (without diabetes), cowritten with another geriatrician, and in a book specifically on the secrets of living long and healthfully with diabetes, coauthored with a diabetologist. And Dr. Colberg has over 57 years of living well with type 1 diabetes under her belt to boot, so she adds both professional and personal experience with aging and diabetes to the mix.

How do we best approach aging with diabetes? Proactively—meaning that we focus not only on managing diabetes in an age-appropriate way but also on preventing and dealing with other diseases or chronic conditions that can cause premature death or limit the quality of life. As Dr. Colberg likes to say, what's the point of living longer if you can't feel your best every day of your life?

LET'S TALK ABOUT GETTING OLDER IN GENERAL

It's common for people to blame all their ills on getting older—even when they're much younger than anyone old enough to see a geriatrician. Achy after sitting too long? Yep, it has to be caused by aging. Middle-age spread? That happens to everyone (and must be caused by aging). In reality, many of these so-called consequences of getting older are actually reversible with lifestyle changes or preventable in the first place. And most are not inevitable.

Both of us have had similar issues. As Dr. Munshi ages, she realizes what her older patients must be feeling. She injured her knee and was having a hard time getting up from a squatting position without pain. And she thought, "Here it goes—this is now lifelong arthritis pain." Then one day, six months later, the pain just disappeared. So her favorite saying to her patients who are recovering from minor or major illness is "This is a speed bump, not the end of the road." Dr. Colberg has had type 1 diabetes for well over half a century and never knows whether to blame her joint aches and pains on diabetes (which makes her more prone to overuse injuries), aging, or true overuse. She has found that given enough time—and often some targeted exercise or physical therapy—she recovers from her joint problems, even though a diabetologist told her that her shoulder issues were permanent. Sometimes, though, it does take years for them to stop annoying her or getting reinjured.

Given that all the cells in our body have a limited life span, it should come as no surprise that the human body does as well. Each cell in every tissue or organ can split and reproduce only a certain number of times before dying, although the types of cells vary in how quickly they turn over. In fact, in the average adult about 330 billion cells get replaced daily, which is about 1% of all your cells. You're constantly sloughing off skin cells, hair, and more. Organs like your liver have a remarkable capacity for regeneration. Overall, in about three months your body will have replaced around 30 trillion cells— about the same number it would take to replace yourself entirely. The biggest component of getting older is the slowing down of your cells' turnover rate, leading to faster aging. External factors like emotional distress and physical trauma, as well as your environment and lifestyle, can negatively affect the generation of new cells and their life expectancy. Your genetics also plays a role in how long you live and how well your body holds up.

From a whole-body perspective, aging is complex and involves a gradual decline in the physiological function of various systems of your body. Nerves transmit signals more slowly; your maximal pulse rate declines; the immune cells decrease in number (and effectiveness); skin cells lose their elasticity; joints become less flexible; bones become less dense and more brittle—you get the picture. On top of all that, diseases and ailments can come along and contribute to worsening health.

It can be difficult at times to determine whether a particular ailment or symptom is due to getting older or to a specific disease process or other factor. For example, you may lose some feeling in your extremities over time. Such losses can certainly be a result of aging, but they can also be due to diabetes (*neuropathy*), medications (such as longtime metformin use), vitamin deficiencies, medical treatments (like chemotherapy for cancer), genetics (tall stature), or other causes.

Whether you can truly ferret out which of your health issues may be caused by the process of aging and which are due to disease is not as relevant as you might think. You just need the best treatments and delaying strategies. If it were possible to prevent all diseases, humans would still die of nothing but old age. What we hope to do is help you manage diabetes and any other health conditions in the right order, with the goal of keeping you from becoming impaired from a preventable or treatable condition or dying prematurely. We also want to help maximize how well you are living—your overall quality of life—for the years you have remaining.

WHO QUALIFIES AS BEING AN "OLDER ADULT"?

Dr. Munshi prefers not to label people as "seniors" because that may include everyone who is 50 and older, depending on the context. Getting an AARP card and the senior discounts that go with it starts at age 55, but you can join the organization at any age without receiving the discount benefits. Medicare currently kicks in for everyone at the age of 65, and those are the youngest people she sees in her clinic at Joslin, with the oldest being 101 at present. She truly believes that you are as young as you feel, though, and she knows firsthand that chronological age does not predict how well someone is living in their later years. More and more adults aged 65 and older are high-functioning individuals treated the same as younger adults in professional and other settings. Over the past 20 years, Dr. Munshi has seen more of the "sandwich generation," which used to be defined as individuals taking care of their kids and their parents but now comprises individuals caring for their parents and grandkids. This change shows that people are living longer and remaining highly functional at older ages.

On the other hand, some people in their 70s, 80s, and 90s have trouble taking care of themselves and doing basic self-care. Those are the individuals whom she considers "senior." Sometimes, it just depends on their mental outlook. Dr. Munshi has two patients aged 85 with very similar medical problems and abilities. One says, "I'm the luckiest person in the world; I have the best doctors and a caring family, and I'm enjoying life the best I can," whereas the other person says, "Why am I even here? Look at how many diseases I have, and I feel like a burden." So much of this is in the attitude!

HOW CAN YOU STAY FEELING YOUNGER?

Picking long-lived parents before you were born would have been helpful to your overall longevity potential, but don't despair if you don't have the best family history of long life. Your genes control no more than 50% of your longevity, while the rest is up to you. A better goal is to live well and feel younger than your actual age for as long as you are alive, and accomplishing that is much more under your direct control. You can start at any age to increase your odds of living longer—and with a stronger body and mind.

From about age 40 to 60, regular exercise was important, along with avoiding gaining too much fat weight, choosing better foods to eat, drinking in moderation only, not smoking, and having regular health checkups and preventative screenings (like colonoscopies, mammograms, and prostate-specific antigen levels for your prostate). Staying active mentally and having a social life were also a part of making sure you were living well and enjoying life.

But now you have hit the big 6–0, and your priorities for the next two decades should change a little. Exercising regularly is still important. But if you haven't already started, you really need to do balance training and resistance workouts to help you retain muscle and stay on your feet. Including these types of exercise sooner than age 60 is more beneficial, but now you really can't ignore them. You may want to avoid losing weight by just dieting—it needs to be combined with exercise so you keep muscle, the good weight, and lose mostly fat, the bad weight—and focus on more than preventing weight gain. Most of the other preventative screenings and recommendations still apply, but you should also start checking your bone health and consider getting vaccinated against pneumonia, shingles, and other pesky illnesses that can damage your health more easily the older you get. It's also time for you to look at how many medications you may be taking to avoid having to take too many.

Once you have made it to 80 and beyond—like so many more people are doing these days, at least before the recent pandemic—you may need to consider additional safeguards to ensure your continued good health. You may need to safetyproof your home to prevent falls or injuries if you do fall. You may need to consider using a cane or a walker if you become unsteady on your feet. But if you have made it this far, you should also keep doing a lot of the same things you have already been doing. Keeping a positive mental outlook and a good attitude toward life can keep you living well for a lot longer, and being proactive about your health is part of that.

We likely don't have all the answers for you—getting older is an individualized journey, and older adults are not just younger adults with wrinkles—but we'll try to guide you down some better paths that may lead to more optimal outcomes for you or for your loved ones as they travel down this road. Taking our advice may not slow the process of aging, but following the actionable items in this book that you find relevant will likely make the rest of your years with diabetes (or any other health condition) as enjoyable and manageable as possible.

HOW LONG WILL YOU LIVE?

Why doesn't everyone live to 100 or beyond since that is closer to the actual capacity of the human body? Accidents aside, it's because most people die from disease although their cells have the capacity to live longer. Even nowadays, the leading causes of death for adults around the world are heart disease and cancer, which are often preventable. The average life span of men and women in the United States is still in the late 70s, with women living at least 5 years longer than men overall. We had been making strides for decades in increasing life expectancy and preventing premature death for both sexes until the recent COVID-19 pandemic reversed that trend, and life expectancy dipped below 80.

It's very likely that your biological age—or how your body is working—is more important to a long life than your actual age in years. If you are 50 years old but have poor health compared to others your age, you are actually biologically older than they are. If you are

80 or beyond and doing well, you may outlive a lot of people you know.

When it comes to the impact of your genes on your longevity, it again bears repeating that your genetics are not your destiny. How well you deal with factors like mental stress has an impact on cellular aging. Being able to control your body's level of inflammation—known to contribute to heart disease, insulin resistance, diabetes, and high blood pressure—can slow how rapidly your cells age. Various tissues in your body and your organs age at different rates, but you can take action to help slow their aging as well. Many of the steps recommended in this book focus on managing those aspects of aging that you can directly affect via what you choose to do and how you live your life.

NO TWO OLDER ADULTS WITH DIABETES ARE THE SAME

So you have diabetes (or prediabetes), and your doctor wants you to manage it. You would think that mentally and emotionally everyone would be the same. But no two older adults face the same set of circumstances when it comes to aging and managing health problems—as a group, older adults are very heterogeneous. For example, if you were diagnosed with either type of diabetes at a younger age, then you might have adapted more easily to making the changes in your daily life that a chronic disease like diabetes demands. But if you developed diabetes just recently or later in life—even in your 80s and 90s—you may be finding it harder to adjust to such changes and understand all the nuances of managing it.

If you live alone, it is even more difficult to take care of your diabetes when you are not feeling well or have other health issues. If you live with someone, then you may have a support system but worry about burdening your loved one; perhaps you're a caregiver yourself. You may live in a community for older adults, in a rehab facility, or even in a nursing home, and your ability to take care of your diabetes may vary based on the setting. In any of these cases, it helps to have more information and another game plan to help you deal with it.

Health status is seldom stable as we get older, and the need or the ability to keep tight glucose levels may change over time for many reasons with advancing age. For example, in older adults with multiple risk factors for experiencing low blood sugar (that is, *blood glucose*), keeping levels on the lower side may be counterproductive. A better goal is aiming for levels that are as good as possible without increasing the risk for any lows at all, which catastrophically can lead to poor balance, falls, decreased thinking ability, and more when you're older. If you're dealing with multiple illnesses or disabilities, your health and wellness goals will definitely need to be individualized to adapt to your changing circumstances. Just aging alone can limit your body's ability to compensate if you get injured or experience organ failure. Your diagnosis and care of any health issues may certainly change with advancing age.

WHY MANAGING DIABETES AND PREDIABETES IS IMPORTANT

While we don't plan on harping on all the potential health complications that can be associated with having diabetes of any type, it is good to understand that it can have a negative impact on your health. For example, people with diabetes (and often even those with prediabetes) can lose muscle mass more quickly over time, have more fat in places around the body where it does the most harm (such as deep in the belly), experience systemic inflammation that increases the risk of heart disease and other blood vessel blockage, have a dysfunctional gastrointestinal tract, lose bone mass more quickly and become frail, develop certain cancers, and end up with cognitive declines, dementia, or Alzheimer's disease. We're not trying to scare you but rather let you know that having diabetes can be a wake-up call to choose to improve your health now—and potentially prevent or delay any and all of these possible outcomes.

WHAT TO EXPECT IN THE PAGES AHEAD

Everyone knows that aging is serious business, but we all also agree that it usually beats the alternative. Although growing older is inevitable, it can be a difficult mental and physical journey for many. If you weren't motivated before to live your best life for as long as possible, you will be once you finish reading this book. You'll learn tips about how to improve your lifestyle and your health in age-appropriate ways, especially with diabetes or prediabetes. If you care for someone else aging with diabetes, you have an invaluable resource at your fingertips. Each chapter outlines what's old, what's new, and how you should approach different areas of health and well-being, including physical activity, diet, mental and brain health, disease prevention, body weight, and much more.

While most books on diabetes focus on its reversal and blood glucose management alone, you're going to be learning more about implementing as many tips and lifestyle changes as possible to better manage your health first and foremost and blood glucose levels second. The innovative steps will help you to accomplish the following:

- Simplify your life with diabetes and avoid low blood glucose
- Change your lifestyle to minimize the highs as well

- Get and stay more physically active in ways that seldom require breaking a sweat or leaving your home
- Lower your insulin needs by reducing inflammation and improving the health of your gut
- Make improvements in meal choices that work for you at your age—without having to completely overhaul the way you eat
- Rev up your brain power, especially if you're starting to feel more forgetful or have problems with managing diabetes on your own
- Learn ways to develop a more positive attitude about aging with diabetes
- Choose the right diabetes and other medications to lower your risk for drug interactions
- Avoid certain cancers, cardiovascular disease, dementia, and other health conditions often associated with getting older
- Have the best body (shape and size) that you can to avoid other health issues, especially those caused by losing muscle and gaining fat
- Live your best life for the rest of your years—even with diabetes

So let's get started and get you on the road to better health, no matter your current age or health status. You've got this!

CHAPTER ONE

Step 1: Change Your Sweetness

When you were diagnosed with diabetes (of any type), or even pre-diabetes, your health care provider probably told you that the most important aspect of managing your diabetes is to learn how to keep your blood sugar (more correctly referred to as *blood glucose*) levels in check. But did you know that you may need to change how you approach this as you get older? No specific number is considered to be "old age"—everyone is a day older today than yesterday. Think of aging as a continuum, and change your thinking and goals to compensate.

With age comes wisdom, or so they say. It is likely you have already encountered a few life-altering events that turned your daily life and focus upside down. When "life happens" and your diabetes management gets temporarily waylaid, do not panic. It is okay to put it on the back burner while you handle other stresses and then focus on your diabetes a bit later. In the meantime, many self-care tips are available to help you manage life and ultimately boost your health and vitality (box 1.1).

You may wonder why this topic is the first of a 10-step action plan to feel more youthful no matter your age. It isn't because desirable blood

> **BOX 1.1**
>
> **Step 1: Change Your Sweetness**
>
> - What's old
>   - Aiming for tight blood glucose management for everyone with diabetes, regardless of age, health status, and goals
> - What's new
>   - Focusing first and foremost on preventing blood glucose lows as you age and simply reducing your time with elevated levels if possible
> - What you should be doing
>   - Working with your health care team to personalize your blood glucose targets depending on your overall health, chance for lows, and more
>   - Allowing your numbers to rise without fear when you are trying to avoid lows because all high numbers are not the enemy—guard against the persistent highs instead

glucose levels are the most important part of aging successfully—although they can help. It is because the aspects of blood glucose management that affect your quality of life—that is, how well you live and how good you feel—may matter more as you reach your golden years than focusing solely on the levels themselves.

WHAT IS BLOOD GLUCOSE?

Glucose, a simple sugar, is one of three *monosaccharides* in your bloodstream. When your body digests food, it breaks it down into more easily absorbed molecules, of which glucose is one. The other two simple sugars are fructose (or fruit sugar) and galactose (part of milk sugar). All sugars are found naturally in foods and drinks, along with *disaccharides* called sucrose (white table sugar), lactose (milk sugar), and maltose (malt sugar) and more complex carbohydrates. Although the idea of having too much sugar in your blood—which is primarily glucose—may frighten you, adequate levels are necessary because your brain and your nervous system use blood glucose as a fuel almost exclusively. Your muscles and other tissues also use glucose for energy.

Blood glucose comes from different sources but mostly from what you eat. Foods rich in carbohydrates like grains, rice, milk, fruit, potatoes, other starchy root vegetables, and corn are released as glucose in your bloodstream after your body fully digests them. Glucose enters your blood after you consume anything—even protein—and is not really a reflection of how much sugar is in your diet. If you do not have diabetes, your blood glucose can rise modestly and temporarily after you eat. Much of the resulting glucose gets used by your brain, nervous system, and active muscles. The rest gets partitioned into various storage areas around your body, primarily your skeletal muscles and liver.

Having high blood glucose levels for too long can cause problems, but so can glucose levels that are too low. It is a fine balancing act that is usually well orchestrated by your liver. After you eat and at times when carbohydrates are abundant, your liver receives a signal to store glucose for later use. When glucose is less available or is being used at a faster rate—such as overnight or whenever you are fasting or engaging in extended physical activity sessions—your liver can release glucose to keep your levels normal. It can do this by either releasing stored glucose or creating new glucose from other sources (through a process called *gluconeogenesis*).

In this book we focus on helping you manage your blood glucose levels as effectively as possible while you are aging with diabetes. Do not be afraid to reassess your goals for diabetes management. As you reach your later years, easing up on your targets for blood glucose levels to make them a little less tight does not mean you're giving up. You are simply adjusting the balance between what is most important for you at a different stage of life. While you may currently think that managing your glucose should be the primary focus of anyone with diabetes, this first step will demonstrate why you should worry less about managing it and more about preventing any and all lows and improving your health in other ways. By following the steps in this book, you will likely experience fewer elevated blood glucose levels without having to put so much effort into managing them, and you will likely need fewer medications.

HOW SHOULD YOU MANAGE YOUR BLOOD GLUCOSE?

One of our primary reasons for writing this book is not only to improve blood glucose levels in people growing older with diabetes but also to get you to a higher level of functioning and the best quality of life possible (box 1.2). We avoid diabetes management plans that can overwhelm—emotionally, financially, or physically. Keeping you safe is the primary concern. Ask why. Why are we chasing after certain numbers? To avoid complications and live a high-quality life. If your treatment becomes too stressful, we are defeating the purpose.

Official guidelines can educate you about how best to manage your diabetes when you get older or are diagnosed with diabetes later in life. One important consideration is whether you are dealing with any other health problems—which gets more likely with age. Juggling more than one health issue can be challenging and complicate your care. In fact, some health problems can make it very difficult for you to care for yourself, and diabetes is one of those chronic diseases

BOX 1.2
Insight from Dr. Munshi

I have seen patients, along with their families, suffer from tremendous stress because their diabetes is not well managed. For instance, one patient had a stroke and was hospitalized for a while before going to rehab. His wife was concerned that he needed to get his blood glucose under control to keep his health from worsening. They were both overwhelmed.

I told them to develop a priority list:

- First, get him up and moving. Physical therapy is very important, and so is mental help in adapting to life after a stroke.
- Then, get his blood pressure under control.
- He should concentrate next on gaining back the weight he lost since weight loss after an illness can cause a loss of muscle in addition to fat. He will need to eat more to regain muscle.
- Once his physical and mental health approach his baseline before his stroke, we can focus on his diabetes and get back to tighter blood glucose levels.

His scenario is similar to what I tell people who must take steroids for their asthma (which end up raising their blood glucose) or anyone newly diagnosed with cancer or experiencing unfortunate social circumstances. Prioritize and simplify. Take care of this new event, and diabetes will still be there to manage more effectively once you're doing better.

---

that requires self-care. Let's say you have a stroke, low vision, or reduced hearing. Any one of these may make it harder for you to monitor your glucose, take prescribed medications, and manage your diet and activity levels.

You may also live alone, in which case you need treatments that are safe and easy to manage by yourself. And while the point of managing your blood glucose levels is to prevent future health complications, getting too low can put you at risk for other issues—some dangerous.

Just imagine if your glucose drops too low and causes you to fall and injure yourself. That is of much more immediate concern than worrying about preventing possible developments in the future.

WHAT TYPE OF DIABETES DO YOU HAVE?

Let's talk about what type of diabetes you have. It is not a new disease. Diabetes mellitus was first noted millennia ago. When your blood glucose exceeds a certain level (usually around 200 mg/dL, or 11.1 mmol/L), your kidneys filter out some of the excess and dispose of it via the urine by pulling extra water out of your bloodstream. Some of the classic symptoms of diabetes—such as frequent urination—are thought to have been first mentioned in writings by an Egyptian physician in 1552 BC. Early physicians named the condition *diabetes*, meaning "siphon," because patients with this disease became emaciated. A Greek physician named Aerates described these individuals as experiencing "the melting down of flesh and limbs into urine" back in 150 AD. The sweetness of the urine from such patients attracted ants, so *mellitus*, meaning "honey," was added to its name in 1675.

Centuries later, in the 1800s, diabetes was still being diagnosed by tasting the urine of ailing patients for sweetness until a chemical test for sugar in the urine was finally developed. It was not until the 1980s that home monitoring of blood glucose using finger sticks and small glucose monitors became more widely available. Nowadays, luckily, we have a variety of testing options to check for excess sugar in the blood and urine, making both the diagnosis and management of diabetes so much more civilized than tasting urine.

In today's world, what diabetes is to an older person and how each individual deals with it depend on many factors. It isn't a one-size-fits-all health condition. The many types of diabetes that exist nowadays can create confusion, and their causes vary, but one thing remains consistently true: how you manage your health must adapt with age, especially if you have diabetes, regardless of the type. Your risk of developing diabetes of any type increases with age, reaching 29.2% if you're aged 65 years or older.[1] Whether you are new to diabetes or a long-time veteran of this disease, you can benefit from the action steps laid out in this book. First, let us review the types of diabetes (box 1.3), how diabetes is diagnosed, and what you generally need to know about its usual treatments.[2,3]

What Is Type 1 Diabetes?

The less common of the two main types, type 1 diabetes is considered to be the result of your own immune cells attacking your pancreas (the organ where insulin is made) and destroying just the beta cells that make and release insulin. The hormone *insulin* carries glucose to all the cells of the body that are sensitive to it, along with amino acids (the building blocks of protein) and fatty acids (that can be stored as body fat). Your main insulin-sensitive tissues are the muscles, the fat cells, and the liver.

The most prevalent symptoms signaling the onset of type 1 diabetes include needing to urinate frequently, being thirsty all the time,

---

Box 1.3
Types of Diabetes and Prediabetes

- Type 1
- Type 2
- Gestational (during pregnancy only)
- Specific types due to other causes (such as pancreatitis or drug induced)
- Prediabetes

and almost continually feeling hungry. Given that the cells in your body that rely on insulin to supply glucose are literally starving to death, that last symptom comes as no surprise. The first two symptoms are related to excess glucose being filtered out into the urine.

What triggers this *autoimmune* response that ends up wiping out your beta cells in your pancreas remains unclear. It may be a combination of environmental and genetic factors that are still being investigated. Regardless of the trigger, after the majority of the pancreatic beta cells have been destroyed, your blood glucose levels rise, and it is a "starvation in the midst of plenty" situation with too much glucose in your blood (even with some being excreted via the urine) and not enough in your muscle and other cells.

If you are an older individual with type 1 diabetes, it is possible that you developed it during childhood (most common) or at any time during your adult life. Since its onset is more common during youth, many who acquire it during adulthood—when its onset is usually slower than that seen in children—are first misdiagnosed with type 2 and only later correctly diagnosed with type 1 (and put on insulin replacement therapies). Since most people living with this type are adults regardless of when their diagnosis occurred, the length of time they may have been dealing with it upon reaching their older years can vary widely.

What Is Type 2 Diabetes?

It is much more likely that you have type 2 diabetes—which used to be called *adult onset* or *non–insulin-dependent*—because 90%–95% of all cases are this type. If you do have this type, you aren't alone. A recent study in the *Lancet* estimated that although 529 million people worldwide had diabetes of any type in 2021, that number could rise to 1.31 billion by 2050—with type 2 diabetes accounting for 96% of cases.[4] If you are included in this group, you were likely diagnosed with type 2 diabetes during middle age or later, even though the current obesity epidemic has made it more common among teenagers. This type is related in large part to an increased level of resistance to insulin, especially in your muscles and liver (although fat cells can also become resistant to its effects).

Type 2 diabetes is related to lifestyle habits that promote insulin resistance and other bodily changes that lead to high blood glucose levels—so, again, it is caused by a mix of environmental and genetic factors. *Insulin resistance* means that you can still make your own insulin (unlike most people with type 1 diabetes), but it does not work well enough to keep your blood glucose within normal ranges. Many with prediabetes (considered the precursor to type 2 diabetes, in which blood glucose levels are elevated but do not reach the "diabetes" level) have insulin resistance but still make enough insulin to get the job done. You develop type 2 diabetes when the amount of insulin your pancreas produces is no longer enough to overcome your level of resistance to it—and your blood glucose levels rise. Most with type 2 diabetes have some beta cell "burnout," which limits how much insulin they can release. The beta cells lose some or all of their ability to produce insulin when exposed to high levels of blood glucose over time, even though they are not completely wiped out, as in type 1 diabetes.

Since many adults with type 2 diabetes do not have to take supplemental insulin, this type is often considered less severe. In fact, if you have read other books on the topic, you may be convinced that this type is completely reversible and much less serious than type 1. Type 2, however, is much more complex because although you may possess the underlying genes for it, a combination of social, behavioral, and/or environmental factors are required for it to manifest. In fact, many people with type 2 these days have no relatives with type 2, but having a parent, sibling, or other close relative with type 2 diabetes definitely increases your risk of developing it.

Many options are available to "reverse" your type 2 diabetes, or at least manage your blood glucose levels effectively. The idea is to lower your insulin requirements: if you can do that, your body may be able to make enough insulin to provide what you need to keep your blood glucose levels in check. You will want to consider engaging in regular physical activity, improving your eating patterns, losing some body fat (especially around your abdomen), limiting your exposure to pollutants, making sure you aren't deficient in key vitamins and minerals, undergoing bariatric surgery, and more. (Even if you have type 1 diabetes and will never be able to get off insulin no matter what you do, these strategies may limit your insulin requirements and make managing diabetes easier.) Also, a whole host of medications are now available that target different underlying pathologies in type 2 diabetes, including the low-level inflammation associated with insulin resistance and many other metabolic diseases. See step 2 for specific information about the medications used to treat diabetes and steps 3 and 4 for some of the changes you can implement toward being active and eating more healthfully to manage your blood glucose levels.

What Is Prediabetes?

A precursor to type 2 diabetes, prediabetes is diagnosed when you have a relative state of insulin resistance. Nearly 100 million American adults are considered to have prediabetes, whether they know it or not.[1] The numbers total 38% if you count all adults but half of everyone aged 65 years and older. Overall, one in two Americans has either some type of diabetes or prediabetes, which is a huge number of people. Worldwide, diabetes and prediabetes are prevalent in all industrialized and developing countries and affect one in two people in China and India as well.

If you have prediabetes, your blood glucose has yet to reach levels high enough to be considered diabetes, but you are at high risk for

22 • AGING WELL WITH DIABETES

tipping the scale in that direction over time. Worse, you can still develop some of the health complications commonly associated with diabetes without ever progressing past prediabetes, including nerve damage in your feet, heart disease, and stroke. The good news is that it may be easier to reverse prediabetes than full-blown diabetes because at this stage you have lost fewer of your pancreatic beta cells that produce insulin. Making lifestyle improvements that lower insulin resistance is most effective in the prediabetes stage or early in type 2 diabetes, and the same changes that help manage type 2 diabetes, such as being more active and eating better, work to manage prediabetes and keep it from progressing.

DIAGNOSING DIABETES OR PREDIABETES

The three main ways to test for diabetes (or prediabetes) involve simple bloodwork (box 1.4). The first lab test requires a blood draw after you have fasted overnight (without eating or drinking any calories) for at least eight hours. The second test, also performed after fasting, involves drinking 75 grams of glucose (a simple sugar, the main one in your blood) and checking your blood glucose response after one and two hours. The third test is newer and involves a small sample of blood—sometimes just a finger-stick sample—that tells you what your average glucose level has been over the last two to three months. While these A1C tests give your health care team varied feedback about what is specifically going on with your body and allow them to best decide how to treat it, any and all of them can be used to diagnose diabetes or a prediabetic state.

Make sure to have your fasting blood glucose levels tested at least annually and get an A1C test as well if possible. The oral glucose tolerance test (OGTT) is better for determining whether your blood

Box 1.4
Tests for Diabetes and Prediabetes and Their Interpretation

- Fasting plasma glucose
  - A blood sample is taken after eight hours of fasting overnight to test glucose in plasma (the clear part of blood with no red blood cells).
  - This is indicative of your level of insulin resistance overnight and in the early morning hours.
  - If elevated, it specifically diagnoses *impaired fasting glucose* (IFG).
- Oral glucose tolerance
  - This involves drinking 75 grams of glucose and monitoring your blood glucose responses over a two-hour period.
  - It indicates your increase in blood glucose following carbohydrate intake.
  - If elevated, it specifically diagnoses *impaired glucose tolerance* (IGT).
- A1C (glycated hemoglobin)
  - A blood sample—venous or fingerstick—is taken to determine how many red blood cells have glucose bound to a part of hemoglobin.
  - It is indicative of your average daily blood glucose levels over the last two to three months (both fasting and after meals).
  - If elevated, it diagnoses diabetes or prediabetes but does not tell you what time of day glucose levels are usually highest.

glucose spikes too high after meals. Diabetes can sometimes be diagnosed when you are experiencing classic symptoms of hyperglycemia and have a random plasma glucose value of 200 mg/dL or higher. These numbers, unfortunately, do not take age into account. Aging itself causes an increase in A1C for various reasons. Certain levels in each test can result in a positive diagnosis (table 1.1).

If you develop diabetes, you may or may not experience any of its possible symptoms. These can result from elevations in your blood

Table 1.1. **Diagnosis of Diabetes Types and Prediabetes**

	Fasting plasma glucose	Oral glucose tolerance test (OGTT)	A1C	Symptoms
Normal	70–99 mg/dL (3.9–5.5 mmol/L)	2-hour value: 139 mg/dL or lower (7.7 mM)	Less than 5.7%	None
Type 1	126 mg/dL and higher (7.0 mmol/L)	2-hour value: 200 mg/dL or higher (11.1 mM)	6.5% or higher	Classic symptoms of hyperglycemia or a random plasma glucose of 200 mg/dL or above (11.1 mmol/L)
Type 2	126 mg/dL and higher (7.0 mmol/L)	2-hour value: 200 mg/dL or higher (11.1 mM)	6.5% or higher	Classic symptoms of hyperglycemia or a random plasma glucose of 200 mg/dL or above (11.1 mmol/L)
Prediabetes	100–125 mg/dL (5.6–6.9 mmol/L)	2-hour value: 140–199 mg/dL (7.8–11.0 mM)	5.7%–6.9%	Usually none

glucose (known as *hyperglycemia*) and include increased thirst, excessive urination, unusual fatigue, blurred vision, unexplained hunger, rapid weight loss, and even slow-healing cuts and infections. When diabetes onset is rapid—which is most common in youths who develop type 1—these symptoms are more likely to occur. Diabetes can also lead to more subtle symptoms or none at all and remain undetected, particularly if you develop either type as an adult. Even though classic symptoms are not always indicative of diabetes and may arise for other reasons—even temporarily due to an illness or the use of certain medications, such as steroids—you are best advised to see a health care provider to check them out.

What should you do if tests indicate that you may have diabetes? Admittedly, it can be confusing because you may meet the levels on one test and not on another. Do you have diabetes in that case? The answer is yes—you only have to meet the criteria of one test. But how your diabetes is managed may vary according to the test that was positive. For example, if you have a high fasting level but your A1C is normal, your doctor may prescribe a medication like metformin, which is the most commonly prescribed drug for people with prediabetes or type 2 diabetes. That medication will help lower your fasting levels. On the other hand, if your blood glucose spikes after you eat (as indicated by an OGTT), you may need a medication that stimulates your pancreas to release more insulin after a meal but not the rest of the time. Definitely talk to your doctor about which medications or lifestyle changes will work best for you depending on how your diabetes is diagnosed.

IS YOUR GLUCOSE TOO HIGH, TOO LOW, OR ON-TARGET?

Diabetes differs from many other chronic health conditions because it's not all about just lowering one number (as in blood pressure) or raising another (as in HDL cholesterol, the good type). Instead, if you have diabetes, both glucose highs and lows can harm you—but not always equally or in the same time frame.

In fact, you should not be afraid to reassess your goals for diabetes management at this stage in the game. When you are reaching your older years, lowering your goals for tight blood glucose management does not mean everyone is giving up on you. It is simply to adjust the balance between the things that are now most important for you at a new stage of life. Blood glucose management is usually the primary focus of people with diabetes, but you may be better advised to worry less about managing it and more about preventing any and all lows and improving your health in other ways. Following the steps in this book will likely lead to fewer elevated blood glucose levels, without having to put much effort into managing them, and lower medication needs.

Keep in mind that it may be harder for you to change your behavior if you have been managing type 1 diabetes for many decades, and it's okay if you feel anxiety regarding letting go. Once you get older, it is helpful to change your perspective from being fearful of high glucose and not so worried about low glucose to almost the opposite. This change in thinking takes time.

It is well established that elevated blood glucose levels over a long period of time can lead to a number of chronic health complications from damage to the major organs of the body, such as the heart, kidneys, eyes, nerves, blood vessels, and brain. Obviously, then, one goal of tightly managing your glucose at certain levels is to decrease the chances that you harm these vital organs. But again, worrying about them as much when you are older may be unnecessary.

You should aim to keep your levels from going and staying too high. Doing so will help you feel better each day, if nothing else. Did you know, though, that once you are older, preventing hypoglycemia—usually considered a blood glucose level below 65 mg/dL, or 3.6 mmol/L—and minimizing how often you go low may need to become your top goal? That is right—preventing lows may be your only glucose goal as you age.

What We Know about Glucose Goals

So what are reasonable blood glucose goals for most adults as they age, and what do we know about setting them?

1. Younger and older adults need different glucose targets.
   - If you are younger, you can expect to live many more years, which increases your risk of developing the complications

that can arise over decades if your blood glucose stays too high.

- Younger adults typically recover from bouts of hypoglycemia without severe consequences, but you may not if you are older.
- On the other hand, if you are already in your 80s or 90s, you will have less to worry about when it comes to potential long-term complications from glucose highs.
- Lows at any age can have a great impact on your current vitality if they cause falls, fractures, a loss of independence, reduced vigor, or a lesser quality of life.

2. Tighter glucose targets often require more complicated diabetes treatment regimens.

- Taking multiple insulin injections at different times of the day or a variety of glucose-lowering pills can be harder to manage.
- Complicated regimens, as well as getting stressed out about managing all the medications and the dosing, may increase your risk of going low.

3. Targets for the older crowd need to vary with the state of their health and their risk for hypoglycemia.

- If you are older but in good health and have few risks as a result of going low, you may need to focus more on keeping your glucose levels in a tighter range to prevent future complications.
- If your health is subpar or you have a greater chance of having lows for any reason, you may need to prioritize your health now by individualizing your blood glucose goals to prevent lows.

Aiming for the Right Blood Glucose Targets

While lows are typically less of an issue if you do not take insulin, studies have shown in people with type 1 diabetes that aiming to

> **Box 1.5**
> **Reasonable Blood Glucose Goals When You're Older**
>
> - Try to aim for an A1C between 6.5 and 8.0% while avoiding overnight lows and extreme highs in particular, especially if your health is declining for any reason.
> - This is the equivalent of an estimated average blood glucose between 140 and 183 mg/dL (or 7.8 and 10.2 mmol/L).
> - Don't depend completely on your A1C as a goal as you age, though. Various conditions, including age itself, anemia, recent infections, hospitalizations, kidney disease, erythropoietin therapy, gastrointestinal bleeding, and more can make A1C difficult to interpret.

keep overall blood glucose averages lower—when measured with an A1C—may lead to more lows. Although most current recommendations are for an A1C under 7.0% (box 1.5), aiming for 6.0 to 6.5% (or below) may be too low when you are older (but fine when you are younger and less concerned about avoiding lows).[5]

Having an A1C that is 8.0% or higher could lead to too much time with elevated blood glucose levels when you're older, even if you have fewer worries about long-term complications. When your glucose stays high most of the time, you can become dehydrated and need to urinate often. Your risk of falling goes up the more times you get up since many older adults get dizzy when rising from bed or have low vision in darker rooms.

HOW CAN YOU PREVENT AND MANAGE GLUCOSE LOWS?

As we said, avoiding lows—especially severe ones—is going to become your number one goal for living long and well with diabetes.

As you age, you have fewer brain cells you can afford to lose from lows. Additionally, going low can be downright unpleasant, especially if you experience the typical symptoms of feeling shaky, having a rapid pulse, sweating excessively, getting light-headed or dizzy, having trouble thinking or experiencing confusion, suddenly feeling extremely fatigued, seeing visual spots, or even passing out. Going low can also increase your risk of falling, fracturing a bone, and ending up in the hospital (box 1.6).

Sometimes symptoms of lows can mimic neurological symptoms or dementia, making them harder to recognize. Hypoglycemia can easily become a medical emergency if you do not have the wherewithal to treat it quickly and effectively. It can be difficult to think straight when your brain is starving for the glucose that normally fuels its cells and helps you make good treatment decisions. Normal cognitive decline may lead you to be more forgetful—and you may not be as on top of taking your medications, dosing appropriately, or monitoring your blood glucose levels. Frequent lows have the ability

---

Box 1.6

When Is Tight Blood Glucose Management Riskier?

- If you are taking medications with a higher risk of hypoglycemia, particularly any type of insulin and/or sulfonylureas
- If you have previously had severe hypoglycemia that required an emergency-room visit or a hospital stay
- If you have memory problems
- If you are physically frail or have mobility problems
- If you have problems with your vision (in particular, issues that can interfere with proper medication dosing or make you more prone to falling)
- If you have a severe illness, such as heart, lung, or kidney disease

to cause mental decline over time, as well as potentially contribute to the onset of dementia.

What Causes Blood Glucose Lows?

It is widely known that insulin users have a greater risk of going low and experiencing severe episodes, especially as they grow older. Studies have shown that people with type 1 or type 2 diabetes start to show symptoms at lower blood glucose levels than people without diabetes, which puts you at higher risk for developing an episode of severe hypoglycemia that you may or may not be able to treat yourself. Worse, you may become even less aware of the drops or lose all your symptoms of going low over time (known as *hypoglycemia unawareness*). Dr. Colberg has a friend with type 1 diabetes who was aware of his lows for 60 years (from the age of 4 on), but his ability to identify lows on his own suddenly disappeared and has been absent for over 20 years. So even if you experience symptoms of lows now, that does not mean you always will.

You may also start to lose some of your brainpower as you age (known as *cognitive impairment*), and this potential for mental decline and dementia has been shown to be more common in people with diabetes. People with diabetes are also more likely to have other health problems as they age, and some of these can have a negative impact on mental and physical abilities and interfere with treating lows.

How to Prevent and Treat Lows

You can take a number of steps to avoid and treat lows and prevent severe ones. Many revolve around changing your medications—both those you take and their doses.

- Always have rapid-acting carbohydrates handy to treat any lows you may experience; glucose (tablets, gels) works fastest, but other sources can treat lows (like table sugar, certain candies, skim milk, and juices).

- If you use any of the oral pills that stimulate your pancreas to release insulin (primarily sulfonylureas), consider switching to another type of medication.
- Many alternative prescription glucose-lowering medications (oral and injected) that do not cause lows are now available and covered by most insurance plans and Medicare.
- If you are on a complex regimen that involves taking insulin, talk to your team about ways you may be able to simplify it to avoid going low.
- If you take insulin, have glucagon available—such as the new nasal formulation that is easy to administer yourself or to have someone give you—for treating severe hypoglycemia.

You may also be taking medications for other health conditions. As discussed later in step 5, it's possible that when you take more than two or three, interactions between their effects can increase your chances of developing bad lows, especially if you take sulfonylureas (like glyburide) or insulin. Talk with your health care team about managing your medications to avoid any possible interactions that can put you at risk for going low.

MINIMIZING GLUCOSE HIGHS

Preventing or experiencing fewer blood glucose highs may follow from the lifestyle changes discussed in the other action steps. Modifying your diet can help. Losing a little bit of body fat and keeping your muscle mass gives you a greater storage capacity for blood glucose out of the bloodstream. Staying active makes your insulin work more efficiently and keeps systemic inflammation in check.

In fact, as you age your health may benefit more from preventing the long-term health issues that can arise from high cholesterol levels or high blood pressure, not just higher blood glucose. That said, spending less time with high glucose levels is still important. In some studies, older adults with more poorly managed blood glucose levels have been shown to be more impaired, with ailments such as hearing loss, poor vision, a history of recent falls (and a fear of falling), and trouble completing the normal activities associated with their daily lives.[3] There is a fine balance between managing blood glucose levels to prevent lows and not running too high most of the time.

Your blood glucose may be elevated in the morning before you eat and spike after meals and snacks during the day. As you age, though, it may be more important to focus on how to prevent your glucose levels from rising dramatically after meals than on your fasting levels. Check step 3 for information on managing those postmeal spikes more effectively by changing what and possibly when you eat.

In addition, several medications used to treat various health problems can raise your blood glucose and make controlling it more difficult. Check with your health care team about what to expect and how to better manage your glucose if you use any of these types of medications:

- Steroids (also called corticosteroids), including local injections for pain relief
- Certain treatments for anxiety, attention deficit hyperactivity disorder (ADHD), depression, and other mental health issues
- Pills for high blood pressure (beta-blockers, thiazide diuretics) or cholesterol (statins)
- Birth control pills (and injections)

- Some treatments for asthma, acne, HIV, and hepatitis C
- Adrenaline (taken for severe allergic reactions)

HOW TO MONITOR YOUR GLUCOSE

Once blood glucose self-monitoring became widely available in the 1980s, the hope of managing glucose levels became a reality. Urine testing for glucose quickly became a relic of the past because it was only slighter better than nothing until a useful testing method came along.

Finger-Stick Glucose Meters

Nowadays, blood glucose meters come in a variety of brands and models, all of which give a single point-in-time reading from a single drop of blood. As for when or how often to check, it is generally helpful to monitor not only first thing in the morning but also before and after meals, around physical activity, and at various other times to confirm symptoms of lows or highs. For Dr. Colberg, who developed type 1 diabetes and went the first 18 years without access to any glucose monitoring, getting her first meter finally gave her to the tools to achieve much more normal blood glucose levels overall.

Even if you do not take insulin, it is still possible for your blood glucose levels to fluctuate when you eat, sleep, exercise, and more. These numbers rarely stay stable all day long, and they are important to check to keep your levels in a desirable range for you. Even just being more active one day than another can potentially have a big impact.

Using your meter can be motivational, especially if your blood glucose goes down when you are active, and that is what you are hoping to achieve. Actually seeing it happen can be very reassuring.

Consider these factors when choosing a blood glucose meter:

- Ease of use and features
  - Evaluate more than one if possible to determine which will be easiest for you to use. Some have bigger numbers that are easier to see, and others provide auditory alerts that tell you when to apply your blood sample and when the check is complete. Choose the one that is best for your needs.
- Cost and insurance coverage
  - Your insurance may cover only certain models or pay for a limited number of test strips per month. Choose a meter that allows you to check your glucose as often as needed. If you have a copay for the test strips, get one that meets your budget.
- Data storage
  - Most meters today store a great deal of information so you do not have to write it down—including times, dates, trends, and more—and others allow you to add data, such as whether you are taking your reading before or after eating or exercise. Many let you store all this information on a computer or mobile app that you can easily share with your doctor and others. Choose the features that make blood glucose management easiest for you.

It is also worth mentioning that although blood glucose meters aren't infallible, poor readings can result from the procedures you use to perform a check. Make sure your fingers are clean before you stick them, warm them up if possible to make your drop of blood flow easier, avoid pricking the callused tops of your fingertips (from checking a lot), and stay hydrated so your glucose levels do not give false high readings.

Continuous and Intermittent Glucose Monitoring

In the past couple of decades, various continuous (and intermittent) glucose-monitoring (CGM) systems have been developed and approved for use. These systems are all minimally invasive, meaning they use a sensor inserted below the skin from 3 days to 6 months. Most of these monitors allow users to obtain a glucose reading every 5 minutes or so, 24 hours a day. People with type 1 and type 2 diabetes can use these devices, as can pregnant women with gestational diabetes (and some people without diabetes). Their main drawback is a lag time that varies from a few minutes up to 20 between the measured glucose (which is sampled between cells in what is called *interstitial fluids*) and the actual blood glucose level.

In some studies, using CGMs resulted in better blood glucose management overall, particularly in youths and adults with type 1 diabetes whose glucose levels are higher (that is, an A1C of 8% or above, or greater than 64 mmol/mol) and in some adults with type 2 diabetes.[6,7] For older adults who are less aware of developing hypoglycemia, using a CGM device may be very beneficial in alerting them to treat lows.[8,9]

Some of the challenges with older adults, however, arise from having poorer hearing, reduced vision, and lesser brainpower. As one older man with type 1 diabetes explained, he can't wear his hearing aids to bed and sometimes doesn't hear the low alerts on his CGM. He is also more easily distracted now and forgets to take his insulin, causing his glucose levels to fluctuate more. In such cases you may need to use a CGM that allows you to share your readings with another family member or friend who can contact you when your levels drop too low. Diabetes technologies are not perfect, though, and CGM usage has some pros and cons (box 1.7).

Box 1.7
What Are the Pros and Cons of CGM Use?

Pros

- Glucose readings are frequent (usually every five minutes) rather than limited in number.
- Alarms can notify you about glucose highs and lows.
- Trend arrows can alert you to impending glucose changes.
- Values can be shared with family members or friends remotely.
- Most devices have small sensors to wear discretely on various areas of your body.
- Costs have come down tremendously, and most are covered by insurance.

Cons

- Sensors are currently still invasive (with a wire under your skin).
- Lag time exists between sensor-measured glucose and actual blood glucose levels.
- Sensors must be changed periodically (most last 7–10 days), and sensors may fail early on occasion and need to be replaced.
- Glucose readings are not always accurate (but neither are fingerstick values).
- Not everyone wants to wear a sensor, and some may become fatigued from too much feedback.
- Alarms can be annoying, and most low alarms can't be silenced.

The Future of Glucose Monitoring and Insulin Delivery

The means to monitor your blood glucose are rapidly changing, and the future for even better methods looks bright. Many groups are working on alternate techniques, including the use of noninvasive and long-term implantable devices. Having the right tools and alarms that can warn you of impending highs and lows can be critical to managing diabetes as you get older.

One particularly exciting development is the automated insulin delivery (AID, or hybrid closed-loop) system, which consists of a CGM, an insulin pump, and a separate device for collecting results and automating the delivery of insulin via an algorithm. For anyone who uses insulin, such a device to completely handle adjusting basal (background) insulin could be immensely helpful in avoiding glucose lows and highs.

At present, all such AID systems approved for use in the United States still require some user input, primarily for meals and physical activities. If or when these systems become fully automated, diabetes management may become much easier, especially if you experience any loss in brainpower or in the ability to make complex decisions about insulin dosing and food intake. Look for these systems to become much more sophisticated and user-friendly as time goes on.

GETTING IT RIGHT

The most important thing to remember is that your health status will continue to evolve as you get older. None of us is going to live forever, but we all want to spend our days with as much vitality and enjoyment as possible. Even if you're in good health and your current goal is to tightly manage your blood glucose levels, you may need to adapt your target numbers over time to changes in your health. Stay open to setting new goals as needed—for blood glucose and other health parameters—to keep up with the circumstances associated with getting older. And have a good network of family, friends, neighbors, or health care providers in place who can help you age backward throughout your later years.

CHAPTER TWO

Step 2: Reverse Your Road to Diabetes

Did you know that you can reverse your direction down the road to type 2 diabetes, prediabetes, and insulin resistance? Whether such conditions are fully reversible (type 2 diabetes and prediabetes) or you would still need insulin (type 1 diabetes), but maybe less of it, you can alter your path toward truly problematic diabetes by getting a handle on the inflammation and insulin resistance that can lead to complications and health problems like high blood pressure and heart disease. And you'll have the added bonus of better overall well-being, more energy, and the ability to enjoy life more.

If you focus on prevention and intervention early on, you will likely have an easier time with your blood glucose management and better health overall since any insulin in your body is going to more efficiently lower your blood glucose levels. In addition, making some easy lifestyle changes will help tamp down inflammation, which is often the culprit in other health conditions (box 2.1).

Regardless of which type of diabetes you have, you can be resistant to insulin whether you make your own, inject it, pump it, or

> **Box 2.1**
>
> **Step 2: Reverse Your Road to Diabetes**
>
> - What's old
>   - Prescribing medications to lower insulin resistance for everyone with prediabetes and type 2 diabetes—and even to some with type 1 diabetes
> - What's new
>   - Using lifestyle interventions to manage and lower insulin resistance and low-level inflammation in the body
> - What you should be doing
>   - Focusing on the lifestyle habits that will actually increase how long you can live well, along with those that improve your blood glucose and level of insulin resistance, lower blood pressure, and benefit your cholesterol levels to achieve better heart health

inhale it (yes, those are all current insulin-delivery options). Just knowing that makes insulin resistance relevant to everyone with diabetes of any type or prediabetes (box 2.2).

WHAT IS INSULIN RESISTANCE?

So you've been told that you have *insulin resistance*. But what does that mean, exactly? To better understand what you're dealing with, think of it as a lock and key. In your body, glucose from the foods you eat and that your liver makes has to get from your blood and into your muscle and fat cells (the main cells sensitive to insulin). In the muscles, glucose gets used immediately for energy to allow your

> **Box 2.2**
> **Insight from Dr. Munshi**
>
> If they are dealing with being overweight or having obesity, I tell patients who are eating unhealthy food or living a sedentary life that their diabetes diagnosis may have increased their functional life span by many years. Why? Because they are now going to do what they should have already done, which is to improve not only their blood glucose but also their blood pressure, cholesterol, joint health, stamina, and overall health. This is a positive way of looking at the reversal of insulin resistance that their lifestyle improvements are likely to result in.

muscles to contract or stored as *muscle glycogen* for later use. The problem is that for muscle and fat tissues, most glucose can't just enter without assistance to open the "door." In other words, glucose needs a "key" to open the door since it's locked.

Whether produced by your pancreas or taken as a replacement, insulin is the hormone that acts as the key that fits into the "lock" (in this case, the insulin receptors on the surface of the cell) to open it and allow the glucose to enter the cells. If you have the key (insulin) but the keyhole on the lock is blocked, the key won't turn when inserted, or you need two or three keys to open one lock, then glucose still can't enter, and you have insulin resistance. In that case you may have plenty of available insulin that just doesn't work as expected. On the other hand, when your insulin works the way it is supposed to—meaning that your cells are sensitive to it—you only need a single key to open each lock and less insulin to lower blood glucose effectively.

When the keys (insulin) and the keyholes (insulin receptors) work well together, the doors for glucose to enter will open, and the levels in your blood return to normal. Otherwise, you end up with too much glucose in your blood and not enough going into your muscle and fat cells.

Your liver is also sensitive to the level of insulin in the blood, which it uses as a signal to know whether to store glucose (as *liver glycogen*) or release some to keep your blood glucose levels in a more normal range at all times. Keeping your liver reacting optimally really helps with leveling out your blood glucose.

HOW IS INSULIN RESISTANCE DIAGNOSED?

If you have insulin resistance (with type 2 diabetes, or even type 1) or prediabetes, you may have no symptoms of it. Severe insulin resistance (which follows chronic inflammation) is associated with a condition called *acanthosis nigricans*, which appears as patches of dark, thick, and velvety skin on your neck, underarms, skin folds, and other areas. This should lead you to be tested for prediabetes and diabetes (see step 1 for the diagnosis of prediabetes). You could have an oral glucose tolerance test (OGTT) or a fasting blood draw administered. A measure called HOMA-IR can assess your level of insulin resistance with your fasting blood glucose and insulin levels as long as you still make your own insulin.

People with type 1 diabetes who must take insulin can also be or become insulin resistant, giving them a "double diabetes" diagnosis.[1] The easiest way to assess insulin resistance with type 1 diabetes is to measure the size of the insulin doses relative to a person's body weight. The more insulin you take relative to your body weight, the more likely you are to be insulin resistant.

WHY DOES INSULIN RESISTANCE MATTER?

As we mentioned, your genes are not your full destiny with respect to your life span. Your body responds to stress—emotional and physical—by releasing stress hormones like *cortisol*, which can affect your body's levels of inflammatory compounds. Inflammation can lead to many metabolic diseases and conditions, including—you probably guessed it—becoming more resistant to insulin.

The levels of glucose in your blood are the result of not only what you take in (food, drink) but also how much your liver releases or stores. During the day (or whenever you're awake and eating) most of it comes from what you consume, particularly foods rich in carbohydrates like grains, starchy root vegetables, fruit, milk, and sugary drinks. We'll talk more about the digestion of foods and blood glucose levels in step 4.

After a meal, your blood glucose levels rise slightly, even if you do not have diabetes, and then drop to normal if you have enough insulin that works like it should. Some glucose from your meals gets absorbed and used by tissues around your body, such as your brain and nerves, along with your active muscles. All insulin-sensitive cells (mainly your muscles, fat cells, and liver) use insulin as a trigger to pick up glucose to use as fuel, although other areas such as your brain can use glucose without insulin. When all systems operational, any excess glucose from your diet gets stored away for later use.

Here's where insulin resistance can be a problem. Any glucose coming from digestion has to be immediately used by cells around your body or stored for later use. To use it or store it in most cells requires insulin. If your insulin fails to work like it should or you do not make or take enough of it, the glucose remains in your bloodstream.

Box 2.3
Who Gets Insulin Resistance?

No matter your type of diabetes—or prediabetes—you can become insulin resistant, and it can happen even if you have neither of these conditions. When you have prediabetes or diabetes, you have a supply-and-demand problem. Although your body can produce insulin, the demand outpaces the supply, partly because of insulin resistance. If you decrease the demand by lowering resistance (i.e., with more exercise or by losing fat cells), then the supply may be adequate to overcome your level of resistance, and you may not need medications to keep your blood glucose in check (making it seem like your diabetes is cured).

Gaining too much weight, living a sedentary life, eating a suboptimal diet, and being mentally or physically stressed can all contribute to insulin resistance. Whether you make your own insulin or have to inject, pump, or inhale extra insulin, that insulin may not work correctly in your body, and you'll require more to do the same job. Muscle, fat, and liver cells can become insulin resistant and lead to higher blood glucose levels. So the potential for becoming insulin resistant is relevant to almost everyone, regardless of whether they have diabetes of any type.

Under normal conditions, insulin binds to its receptors on muscle and fat cells (box 2.3). If you have type 2 diabetes or prediabetes, insulin may be abundant but not that effective (think back to the lock and key mechanism). People with type 1 diabetes have to take supplemental insulin and worry about dosing with the correct amounts. No matter what type of diabetes you have, excess blood glucose that can't enter cells can lead to damage over time—to your blood vessels, your kidneys, your nerves, your eyes, and more. Keeping your blood glucose levels closer to normal helps limit the potential for such health problems over time, and who doesn't want to stay healthy?

WHAT ELSE AFFECTS INSULIN USE?

In addition to insulin failing to work correctly, it's also possible that your pancreas just isn't making enough of this hormone, regardless of your type of diabetes. As you learned, in people with type 1 diabetes, the beta cells of the pancreas have been wiped out by their own immune system. In type 2 diabetes, having to produce so much extra insulin over time to overcome insulin resistance leads to an accumulated loss of insulin-producing beta cells (even without the immune system attacking them). In fact, by the time you were diagnosed with type 2 diabetes, you had already lost some of your ability to make insulin, and you were certainly no longer producing enough to overcome your resistance to it.

Your doctor may have prescribed medications to stimulate your pancreas to make more insulin (like sulfonylureas), or you may have been taking insulin to supplement what you lack. Other medications lower blood glucose in other ways (some lower insulin resistance), but not by specifically causing the release of more insulin.

What's even more interesting is that changing your lifestyle—including your physical activity, your eating habits, your stress-management methods, and your quality of sleep—can match or exceed the impact of taking medications to lower your blood glucose levels. If insulin resistance is the main problem and you are still making your own insulin, improving your lifestyle may reverse type 2 diabetes or prediabetes, particularly if you haven't had either condition for too long. If you have type 1 diabetes and have no choice but to take insulin, you can at least get by with lower doses and reduce your risk of low blood glucose from excess insulin.

Losing some weight often improves how well insulin works. Studies have shown that when healthy people carrying some extra weight change their lifestyles to result in moderate weight loss, they can enhance their insulin sensitivity and lower their state of systemic inflammation.[2] For most adults with prediabetes or type 2 diabetes, the goal is to lose 5%–7% of their body weight, which can dramatically increase their insulin sensitivity. That's only 10–14 pounds if you weigh 200 pounds or 12.5–17.5 pounds if you weigh 250. Now we recognize that not all weight loss is equally good, and we'll talk more about how to lose the right type of weight (if you need to) in step 6.

HOW CAN YOU LOWER INSULIN RESISTANCE?

The good news is that you can galvanize any insulin that you make or take to work better in your body, benefiting your health tremendously. We mentioned lifestyle changes in passing, but let's spend a little more time on why those help and which you should consider trying.

The Impact of Physical Activity

One of the most important ways to lower insulin resistance is with physical activity. Keeping physically fit is critically important, and it's also one of your best bets when it comes to improving how well you age, whether you can live on your own, and how long you live.

Being active has a great impact on insulin because your muscles are the main place where you store excess glucose and carbohydrates. Think of your muscles as a big storage tank for glucose. If your muscles fill up and reach their capacity to hold excess carbohydrates, they become less sensitive to the insulin in your body. In that case your pancreas has to make and release more insulin to do the same job (or you'll need higher insulin doses if you take it), and at some point you may exceed your ability to increase the amount of insulin adequately. So what you really want to do is keep that "glucose tank" large enough to store excess glucose and empty some of it out every day through exercise. Resistance exercise (using resistance bands, weights, or body-weight exercises) is particularly good for building or strengthening muscles and enlarging the tank, and both that type and other forms of exercise can keep the tank ready to accept more glucose. We'll talk a lot more in step 3 about what types of physical activity you should consider.

Why Weight Loss Can Help

The other main cells in your body that insulin affects are your fat cells, the place you store excess fat for later use. In a famine your fat cells can serve you well, but nowadays most of us boast more stored fat than we'll ever need or have the chance to use up. When you gained extra weight, it's likely that your body put some of it not only in fat cells but also in your muscles. In fact, when you gain a lot of fat, your fat cells become too full to accept more (making them insulin resistant), and excess fat ends up in many places that it really shouldn't—including in your pancreas, in your liver, and deep in your abdominal cavity around your organs (*visceral fat*)—and this extraneous fat can interfere with your metabolism and how well your insulin works. This is why losing even a modest amount of body weight, particularly from around your waist, improves your blood glucose levels.[3]

When your muscles are resistant to insulin, your fat cells can usually still store fat when excess glucose is converted into fat—up to a point. Fat cells can also become resistant to insulin when they get stuffed full of stored *triglycerides* (the storage form of fat in your body). When the foods you eat spike your blood glucose because you're insulin resistant, you can end up with more fat in your fat cells that eventually becomes stored in your liver, pancreas, and other internal organs.

Yes, you read that right. You can end up with extra fat in your liver and other organs from being insulin resistant. This matters because your liver in particular ensures you have enough glucose in your bloodstream at all times, storing glucose after meals and releasing glucose when you haven't eaten recently or are exercising. If your liver becomes too fatty, it can become insulin resistant as well. An insulin-resistant liver can release too much glucose overnight and make your morning numbers too high. Losing some weight, especially through physical activity, can remove some of the metabolically disruptive visceral fat both inside your abdomen and your liver.[4]

Other Ways to Rev Up Insulin Action

Insulin resistance is a fluid state, not a static one, meaning that you have the power to change how insulin works in your body. Being more active and losing weight are far from the only factors that can make an impact on the amount of insulin you need. Working to improve as many of these separate influences, listed here along with each step addressing them, on your body's insulin action as possible may vastly improve your diabetes management:

- Managing your blood glucose levels with fewer fluctuations (step 1 and many others)
- Reducing systemic inflammation (step 2)
- Getting regular physical activity of various types (step 3)
- Gaining or maintaining your muscle mass (step 3)
- Eating more fiber and fewer highly refined foods (step 4)
- Eating a healthy breakfast every day to break your fast (step 4)
- Taking in less coffee and caffeine (step 4)
- Taking medications that lower insulin resistance (step 5)
- Losing some extra weight, especially that stored in your liver (step 6)

48 • AGING WELL WITH DIABETES

- Reducing mental stressors, depression, and anxiety (step 7)
- Getting more and better sleep (step 8)
- Managing your physical stressors, such as illnesses, infections, exhaustion, and more (step 8)
- Treating sleep apnea effectively (step 8)
- Decreasing blood levels of cortisol (step 8)

WHAT IS INFLAMMATION AND WHY DOES IT MATTER?

While insulin resistance has been associated with many different metabolic health problems, including obesity, heart disease, high blood pressure, and type 2 diabetes, it's also associated with something called low-level *systemic inflammation*.[5] We've mentioned it in passing multiple times already, but let's talk more about what causes it and why it matters.

Your immune system is quite complex and comprises various types of cells—like macrophages, B cells, and T cells—that are constantly working to defend your body from pathogens and even your own cells when they mutate. Mental and physical stress, infections, and certain chronic diseases can shift your immune system into a *proinflammatory* state. When this happens, your immune cells always remain alert and ready to create inflammation to respond to any bodily changes. Keeping the body safe is logical, but this state is often too much of a good thing and sometimes occurs when you really do not need it.

We know that the body responds to stressors by releasing hormones that prepare us to defend ourselves. For example, when a zebra sees a lion, this "fight or flight" response enables it to run away. That involves the activation of the *sympathetic nervous system*, the one that sets everything in motion for our survival. We are no longer outrunning lions, but when we hear distressing news or think about stressful social events, we create the same neural and hormonal response—and besides being unnecessary, this can harm our bodies long term by increasing insulin resistance and systemic inflammation.

In fact, systemic inflammation can become chronic in response to things like infections, trauma, reduced blood supplies (due to narrowed arteries), a leaky gut (more on this in step 4), and some autoimmune disorders. Inflammation can also be caused by an unhealthy diet, excess body fat, and a sedentary life. It has been established that localized inflammation as a result of immune cell dysfunction affects the beta cells of the pancreas in type 1 diabetes, destroys those cells, and leads to insulin deficiency. Some have hypothesized that a leaky gut may herald the onset of both main types of diabetes and that lifestyle changes may have a positive impact on their development and management.[6]

In the case of type 2 diabetes, insulin resistance is usually a feature of the disease, and systemic inflammation is thought to be an underlying cause of the altered insulin action (rather than insulin resistance causing inflammation). Elevated levels of the hormone *cortisol*, which is released by physical and mental stressors, are often found with insulin resistance and underlying inflammation and may even contribute to fat weight gain.

Acute inflammation can be a good thing, as it can help the healing process. Think of the swelling around your ankle if you twist or sprain it. It lasts for only a short time (hours to days or weeks) and increases blood flow and healing processes in the injured area. On the other hand, *chronic inflammation*, which can last for months or years and has no specific target, can lead to unhealthy metabolic conditions. Its extent and impact vary with the cause, but generally, it lasts until your body can repair and overcome any damage.

What Results from Chronic Inflammation?

In many cases, chronic inflammation can cause diseases that can lead to your early demise. In fact, the World Health Organization ranks chronic diseases as the greatest threat to human health. Many people already have inflammation-related diseases, and over half of all Americans have at least one (and many have more than that).[7] Some have even speculated that heart and blood vessel diseases are fully caused by inflammation, not elevated blood cholesterol levels.[8] A decade ago, nearly 60% had at least one chronic health condition, 42% had more than one, and 12% of adults had five or more. Around the globe, an estimated three in five people who die each year succumb to the health impact of a chronic inflammatory disease. Here's a short list of some of those diseases:

- Cardiovascular diseases, including heart disease, heart attack, stroke, and heart failure
- Obesity and being overweight
- Chronic respiratory disorders like chronic obstructive pulmonary disease (COPD)
- Diabetes
- Cancers
- Arthritis and joint diseases
- Allergies and asthma

In terms of number of deaths, cardiovascular disease leads the pack, followed closely by cancer. The third in line is COPD, including emphysema.

How Do You Know If You Have Chronic Inflammation?

It is possible to measure the levels of certain inflammatory compounds in your blood, such as *cytokines*, that show you have inflammation. They are small proteins (called *peptides*) that all cells in your body make to protect themselves, and they include substances like interleukins, interferons, tumor necrosis factors, certain growth factors, and cellular-stimulating factors. Your immune system produces these to help cells communicate with one another, but they can also have a direct impact on your central nervous system, muscle, bone, and other tissues.

The best recent example of the negative impact of too many cytokines came early in the COVID-19 pandemic, when people were experiencing "cytokine storms" leading to severe organ damage and cellular destruction. Many people with diabetes were the most likely to die in the early days of COVID-19 because we had yet to figure out how to control the cytokine release—which can be accomplished using corticosteroids. By way of example, Dr. Colberg's older sister-in-law, who has type 2 diabetes, got hit early with a COVID-19 infection before the advent of the vaccines for it and nearly died. She had to be treated with steroids to prevent further lung damage, which boosted her blood glucose up over 500 mg/dL and led to her requiring insulin for a while to manage her diabetes after her release from the hospital.

Although measuring for elevated inflammatory markers is a more objective way of telling whether you have inflammation, including C-reactive protein (CRP) released by the liver, most health care providers do not routinely check for them during office visits, and there are few prescribed medications to treat them.

You may want to be on the lookout for certain symptoms associated with chronic inflammation. Some of the more common ones include the following:

- Body and muscle pain
- Chronic fatigue
- Insomnia

- Mood disorders, including depression and anxiety
- Constipation, diarrhea, and acid reflux
- Frequent infections
- Weight gain or weight loss

As you can see, many of these symptoms are very general and potentially applicable to other health conditions, so none of these alone lead to a diagnosis of chronic inflammation.

What Raises Your Risk for Chronic Inflammation?

Some of the risk factors for having chronic inflammation are within your control, while others are not. Getting older is associated with having higher levels of several inflammatory molecules. Why this occurs is not fully understood, but it could be related to the energy-producing parts of your cells (the mitochondria) failing to work properly or free radicals (that is, unstable molecules that contain oxygen and that easily react with other molecules in a cell) building up over time. Fat tissue can secrete its own inflammatory markers, so gaining excess fat weight—especially deep in your abdomen— often causes higher levels of inflammation. Highly processed diets are associated with producing more pro-inflammatory molecules, especially in individuals who are overweight or have diabetes. This may be associated with being deficient in vitamins and minerals, which contributes to the development of oxidative stress and chronic inflammation. Not surprisingly, cigarette smoking reduces your number of anti-inflammatory molecules and induces inflammation, and excess alcohol use also leads to inflammation. Even going through menopause (for women) or "andropause" (for men), when levels of sex hormones like testosterone and estrogen decrease, can result in a greater release of several pro-inflammatory markers. In addition, any stressors, be they physical or mental, can produce inflammatory markers, and stress can cause sleep disorders or disturbances that also boost chronic inflammation. Even doing shift work overnight often contributes to higher levels of systemic inflammation.

How Can You Lower Your Inflammatory State?

Unbeknownst to you, your body is constantly producing unstable molecules called *oxidants*, also known as *free radicals*. Your body's enzyme systems stabilize these oxidants by "borrowing" electrons from nearby molecules. The downside to this natural occurrence is that taking electrons from other areas can damage cell proteins and genetic materials (DNA and RNA), making your cells more vulnerable to cancer and inflammation. What can you do to fight back? Your best defense is to make health-enhancing lifestyle choices (box 2.4).

Box 2.4
Fighting Inflammation Naturally

When your liver becomes insulin resistant, the elevated blood fats and cholesterol levels that can result can contribute to the development of heart disease. Eating foods high in refined (simple) carbohydrates and other highly processed foods can lead to more liver fat. You can lower inflammation and improve metabolic health by making better food choices, such as eating whole grains, fruits and vegetables, beans, and lean protein. Eliminating processed foods (think anything that is prepared and sold in a box) and increasing fiber intake and adopting a more active lifestyle are likely the two most important changes you can make to lower systemic inflammation and the risk of developing all sorts of metabolic diseases. Taking steps to minimize stress, such as meditating or doing yoga or getting outside for even short bursts of time each day, can contribute to your overall well-being.

Physical Activity

Being physically active enhances your body's natural free radical–fighting ability. The use of oxygen during exercise produces these oxidants, and your body responds by improving its ability to squelch them all the time—which is likely why regular physical activity is associated with so many health benefits and fewer chronic diseases. For example, storing extra fat in the liver may contribute to low-level inflammation, which can lead to the development of insulin resistance, diabetes, heart disease, and other metabolic disorders. Exercise helps get rid of some of the excess fat deposited in your liver, which then fights insulin resistance and can leave you healthier in the process. Much more is to come about the impact and benefit of being more active in step 3.

Dietary Improvements

Your dietary choices also have a large impact on your low-level inflammatory state. You may have heard about antioxidant supplements and anti-inflammatory diets. It's easier to know what foods are inflammatory than what are not. For instance, we know that eating a lot of highly processed foods—those usually made with white flour, white sugar, excess sodium, and less healthy fats—can increase inflammation. These compose most of the fast food that Americans routinely eat, unfortunately. These dietary choices are likely to cause blood glucose levels to spike after eating (even if someone does not have diabetes).

Many fast or highly processed foods are high in calories and low in the essential vitamins and minerals that make your metabolism work efficiently. Processing and refining foods too heavily takes out the good stuff, although whether they taste better or worse is a matter of preference. To help lower inflammation, avoid eating highly processed foods and beverages, particularly those containing high-fructose corn syrup, white sugar, white flour, or manufactured trans fats.

Because many diabetes-related health complications are likely related to unchecked oxidative stress in various tissues and organs, eating foods containing more antioxidant power (like berries, seeds, and nuts) that can lower inflammation will help. Focus on eating minimally processed, high-fiber, plant-based foods—that is, most fruits and vegetables, whole grains, legumes, nuts and seeds, and lean protein sources (like egg whites and whey protein)—and other things known to reduce inflammation, such as vinegar, fish oil, tea, and cinnamon. We'll talk a lot more about the best food choices in step 4.

Dietary Supplements

While we are not trying to lead you down the path of taking a lot of dietary supplements—because they are largely unregulated by the US Food and Drug Administration and you never really know what you're getting in most of them—numerous studies have shown the benefit of certain vitamins (such as vitamins C, D, and E and beta-carotene) and minerals (zinc and magnesium) when it comes to lowering chronic inflammation.[9,10] For example, your health care provider may prescribe a fish oil supplement or select vitamin(s), particularly those that people with diabetes are more likely to be lacking. And you can always naturally spice up your foods with spices known to have anti-inflammatory properties, such as turmeric, ginger, and garlic.

Making the Best Choices

Finally, even with all these steps it can be difficult to maintain a healthy diet and exercise routine all the time. Once in a while, enjoying something that is not the best for you doesn't hurt your body permanently as long as you are generally following a healthier lifestyle. Obsessing about it and feeling guilty can only make stress worse—and you should know now what too much stress can do. We'll talk much more about managing mental stress in step 7.

CHAPTER THREE

Step 3: Stand Up and Stride Away

Although older age is considered a time of disability and illness for many, most of the decline with aging likely comes from disuse rather than age alone. You'll do better by being adaptable and keeping on the move in any and every way possible. This may be listed as the third step, but both of us agree that it's critical and one of the most important things you can do for your health and well-being.

Engaging in regular exercise does not mean you're doomed to 30–60 minutes of daily sweating at a gym. Even if you're in a wheelchair or using a cane or walker, you can easily increase your daily movement and gain many health benefits. Just 5 minutes of walking or other physical movement three times a day can be an excellent starting point—and you don't even have to leave home to do it.

The more able-bodied among us can benefit from cross-training, strength building, and balance exercises to enhance fitness, avoid injury, and prevent falls. Even working on your posture is important. We'll cover all these activities in this chapter and discuss why you should remain as physically active as you can possibly be through the end of your life, regardless of your current fitness level (box 3.1).

Box 3.1
Step 3: Stand Up and Stride Away

- What's old
  - Growing older and becoming disabled and blaming it on normal aging rather than disuse
  - Believing that going to the gym, lifting weights, and doing other strenuous activities are only for young people
  - Getting overuse and other injuries and stopping physical activity
- What's new
  - Focusing on physical activity as a means to both prevent disability and to slow normal declines with aging
  - Working out appropriately to avoid overuse injuries
- What you should be doing
  - Working on becoming and staying as physically active as you can in any and every way possible
  - Including various types of physical activity every week to enhance your longevity and your quality of life
  - Exercising smarter and allowing yourself enough time to recover to avoid injuries

WHAT CAN PHYSICAL ACTIVITY DO FOR YOU?

Think about what you really want for the rest of your life. Is it just a longer life you want, or would you prefer to live well and feel better until the end of your days? Adding more years plagued by debilitating illnesses, immobility, or a loss of independence is not what most people desire. On the other hand, feeling well and having the energy to do what you want for as long as you live is truly priceless. Let's talk more about what being active can do for your body and your mind.

Physical Activity Can Prolong Your Life

Did you know that sitting around all the time actually increases your risk of dying early? Studies have shown that when you're older, even engaging in daily activities like volunteering, walking, and chores around the house and yard for an hour or more significantly lowers your risk. Generally, the more active you are, the more benefits you receive when it comes to living longer.

As an exercise physiologist, Dr. Colberg knows how important physical activity is to longevity. But an even better reason to move your body has more to do with the quality of your life than your longevity. Being inactive is the real reason most people experience more fatigue and feel less energetic as they get older, not aging alone. Declines in your energy levels with each passing year are far from inevitable.

If you started becoming more active in your middle adult years, you're more likely to be active and independent in your later years. Both of us know for a fact that exercise is the best "medicine" you can take to prevent debilitating diseases and enjoy a better quality of living throughout your later years.

What can physical activity specifically do for you and your health? In addition to adding some pep to your step (so to speak), staying active lowers your risk of heart disease and helps keep your blood pressure in check. It ensures your muscles remain bigger and your bones stronger. You'll have a lower chance of getting certain cancers—including colorectal, prostate, and breast—and an easier time keeping your blood glucose levels where you want them to be. In fact, if exercise were available in pill form, it would undoubtedly be the best medicine you could ever take for your health. Alas, there is no such thing (but rest assured that researchers have looked into developing an exercise "pill").

Exercising Bestows Many Additional Health Benefits

We're just getting started on the benefits. Aging undeniably causes your body to change over time, independent of disease, even if you remain physically active. We all know that diabetes, especially when not well managed, can lead to health complications, but even those can be hard to differentiate from aging effects. For instance, anyone can develop *peripheral neuropathy* (loss of sensation in your hands and/or feet), especially if you're a tall person or undergo certain cancer treatments. Much of what people attribute to getting older—such as muscle atrophy or a loss of flexibility in joints—results from not using your muscles, not just aging. We used to think that greater insulin resistance was practically inevitable with getting older due to age-related declines in muscle mass, but now we know that older athletes are as insulin sensitive as younger individuals who are physically active. In fact, master athletes have better insulin action than people of any age who are sedentary and either of normal weight or obese.[1] Thin, sedentary people can end up insulin resistant due to a loss of muscle from both aging and inactivity.

Staying active can also benefit your mind in so many ways. Your feelings of overall well-being will likely improve, you'll feel less stressed, you'll more easily overcome mild and moderate depression, and your risk of developing Alzheimer's and other forms of dementia may be cut in half. You're also less likely to experience brain *atrophy* (shrinkage), or at least will slow the rate at which you lose brain cells over time. Exercising increases your blood flow, delivering oxygen to critical regions of your brain (like the *hippocampus*) associated with memory and other functions. Wouldn't you like to improve how well your brain works? In addition to preventing or slowing the onset of dementia, with regular activity you may be able to regain some of what you've already lost when it comes to your mental functioning. What's more, regular exercise may prevent your gut from becoming "leaky," which will greatly enhance your health (see more on the potential impacts of a leaky gut in the next step).

What about sleeping? As you get older, you may find that you're having more trouble falling asleep and staying that way—both how long and how well you sleep can be affected—and increasing your total activity will generally improve your shut-eye time (you'll read more on improving sleep in step 8). Improved sleep enhances your diabetes management, and it also serves to just make you feel happier in general. Joint pain can also keep you awake at night, and as long as you don't overdo it too often, your arthritic joints should actually improve when you're active, making it easier to sleep well.

WHAT IF YOU'VE BEEN INACTIVE?

We both always say that it's never too late to start being more active. You can get more fit by doing anything and regain at least some of any fitness you've lost. Those who start out at the lowest levels of fitness have the most to gain from doing the least—meaning that you'll see big increases in your fitness levels as soon as you start compared to someone who has already been active. Even people who were inactive through their middle-age adult years can still add years to their lives by exercising as they get older.[2] More importantly, getting active at any age will help ensure that any years you have remaining are lived as well as possible. Staying inactive is one of the most quality-of-life-destroying things you can possibly do to yourself—and it's completely preventable with increased physical movement. If you don't want to age prematurely or suffer from unnecessary debilitating illnesses, now is the time to get more active and reverse any downward slides in your health (box 3.2).

> **Box 3.2**
>
> **Preventing and Slowing Aging and Disease with Physical Activity**
>
> Here's what being active can do for various parts of your body and your health:
>
> - **Muscles:** build muscle mass, prevent or slow the loss of muscle over time, increase strength, enhance endurance, and improve the ability to store carbohydrates
> - **Heart:** prevent heart disease, possibly reverse some plaque formation and blockage in arteries, lower resting blood pressure, improve heart strength, and enhance blood flow to the rest of your body
> - **Metabolism and hormones:** raise metabolic rate, enhance energy levels, burn calories, improve use of blood glucose, prevent type 2 diabetes, reverse prediabetes, and increase *libido* (sex drive)
> - **Bones:** prevent some loss of bone minerals, increase bone density, lessen symptoms of arthritis in joints, and lower your risk of bone fractures and falls
> - **Brain and mental health:** feel better and more optimistic, improve memory and learning skills, prevent or slow onset of dementia and/or Alzheimer's disease, lower depression and anxiety, and improve how well you sleep
> - **Longevity:** lower your risk of dying from any cause (including from various cancers and cardiovascular diseases) and increase your life span
> - **Quality of life:** improve your ability to take care of yourself and live independently, keep you mobility and ability to do things you enjoy, and enhance how well you can live and feel while alive

It's really undeniable that one of the most important aspects of improving health overall—and not just managing your diabetes better—is moving your body in various ways on a regular basis. Physical activity has so many health benefits. Want to lower your resting blood pressure? Exercise. Trying to keep your cholesterol in check?

Exercise. Want to keep your heart healthier, your lung function as efficient as possible, and your muscle mass bigger? Exercise.

We all lose muscle mass as we age—even if we're active—but regular activity can help you keep your existing muscle mass toned and slow down how quickly you're losing it. Just being active can help you feel energetic instead of tired all the time. To keep as much muscle as possible, consider doing resistance training at least twice a week. You can use light weights or a resistance band. Even using your own body weight as resistance can be a great exercise. Also try to get in some aerobic activities almost daily. These include walking, stationary cycling, swimming, dancing, and others. They'll really help you keep your blood glucose in check and keep your heart and lungs working better for you.

Honestly, just getting even a little bit fitter than you are now can greatly enhance your metabolism and get your insulin working much better to manage your blood glucose (box 3.3). It's just a side benefit that you can lower your risk of so many other health problems by reducing your insulin resistance, lowering that systemic inflammation

---

Box 3.3
Insight from Dr. Munshi

My favorite quote is "All the numbers I see from your blood test makes me feel good about your health, and exercising regularly will make you feel better and healthier."

Also, as a geriatrician I have observed that exercise is the only fountain of youth. When I see older healthier people in their 90s, they all are physically healthy and active. Some of these amazing individuals tell me that their secret is "to eat moderately, stay physically active, and keep a positive attitude in life." I know that is some of the best advice. I try to incorporate it into my own life and pass it on to my patients.

we talked about in the last step, and keeping all those preventable diseases at bay. Your body weight matters much less when you're active because it's possible to be "fit and fat" and live pretty well, but being active will still likely lead you to lose some body fat while gaining some muscle.

We have to advise you that when you've been inactive—no matter for how long—it's best to start back slowly and progress the same way. Doing too much on one day may make you weary and achy the next, which may keep you from exercising again. Listen to your body, but persist. Another of Dr. Munshi's favorite sayings is "It didn't happen yesterday and doesn't need to go away tomorrow." But you do need to start working on it, and today is a good day for doing that. This applies to your unfitness, sedentary lifestyle, extra body weight, and even less healthy eating patterns.

WHAT SHOULD YOU KNOW ABOUT MUSCLES AND AGING?

We've already mentioned how exercising helps build muscle mass and prevent or slow its loss over time and that having more muscle mass ensures greater strength, more endurance, and the enhanced storage of excess carbohydrates. What you may not know is why all this is true.

Muscle Fiber Types

The purpose of your muscles is to cross joints and allow you to move those joints. The muscles around your body are composed of many different types of muscle fibers, ranging from slow twitch to fast twitch. The "twitch" refers to how quickly the fibers contract to create movement around joints. Think of them as existing in a full continuum from slow to fast twitch, with a limited ability to change types. (What you have in your body is largely genetically predetermined by your ancestors.)

Slow Twitch

The *slow twitch* fibers are, not surprisingly, slow to contract but also fatigue-resistant. You use these fibers to stand or sit upright and maintain your posture. Imagine how hard it would be to engage in daily life activities (including sitting and holding your seven-pound head straight up) if those fibers tired easily. These fibers are largely *aerobic*, meaning they use the oxygen supplied by your blood to convert fuels into usable energy for muscle contractions. You always have some level of contraction going on when you're awake and upright; without these muscle fibers your body would be as floppy as a rag doll.

Fast Twitch

While there are some intermediate fibers as well, on the other end of the continuum are the *fast twitch* fibers. You recruit them into action anytime you need to create a powerful movement. Think of jumping, sprinting, or lifting a heavy item. Most of the time we don't need to rely on these fibers. Just walking around slowly doesn't require their help in most cases. The downside of these fibers is that they run out of energy and tire really quickly. Their main fuel is *anaerobic*, meaning that they create energy without oxygen, such as from carbohydrates stored in muscles (glycogen). You can't use glycogen exclusively in this manner without ending up with a buildup of lactic acid (think of the "burn" in your muscles during heavy work).

As the amount of power you need to create increases, you first recruit the slow, then the intermediate, and then the fast fibers sequentially, as needed. These fast fibers deteriorate the most quickly over time, especially when they aren't used much or at all on a daily basis. It's completely true in this case that if you don't use them, you lose them. If you're on extended bed rest or in a wheelchair, you're losing these fibers in your active muscles even more quickly.[3] That's the primary purpose behind resistance training—to use and challenge these faster fibers so you can retain them as you age.

Muscle Fibers and Muscle Glycogen Use

When it comes to your blood glucose, think of your muscles as a big glucose storage tank. Your goal—if you want better diabetes management—is to keep that storage tank as large as possible and always partly empty. How do you achieve these two goals? First, to work on the size, since you now know that you're losing some muscle mass with each passing decade (starting around age 25), you have to recruit those faster fibers that you lose with disuse. This may involve doing some moderate or heavy resistance training or harder aerobic workouts (if you can). Second, to keep the "tank" always somewhat empty and ready to accept more carbohydrates from the foods you eat, you have to do some aerobic activities that are moderate or harder in intensity. Slow walking, while good for many other reasons, uses little muscle glycogen. You have to pick up your pace from time to time to recruit enough of the intermediate and faster fibers to use more glycogen.

WHAT ARE THE RECOMMENDED TYPES OF PHYSICAL ACTIVITY?

There's no doubt that you want to live well and retain your ability to move and do everything you want to every day of the rest of your life. At some point, physical activity migrates from daily gym workouts, sports, and other activities to the more functionally oriented. What do you need to do to be able to live independently? Are there exercises that can make getting up from the sofa easier and allow you to stand up from the toilet on your own? While such scenarios may be a long way down the road of life for you personally, it's never too early to start working on retaining your ability to care for yourself and to live on your own—and that almost always involves some regular exercise training.

Daily Movement

For starters, to enhance how long and how well you live, you should participate in as much unstructured daily movement as possible. That means being active all through each day in any way you possibly can, including standing up more. Think about how to increase your daily movement doing anything, even if it's just taking "activity breaks" to keep from sitting continuously for long periods of time.[4] If you're unable to be on your feet much or at all, there are alternative activities you can try while seated. If you miss your planned activity on any given day, try to make up for it with additional unstructured physical movement, such as taking more steps overall. By just being more active, you can dramatically improve your physical and mental fitness and your overall health.

Planned Activities

In addition to maximizing your daily movement, consider doing at least four types of planned activities on a weekly basis. All of these exercise training modalities will help you maintain your ability to complete the activities of daily living:

1. Endurance (aerobic)
2. Resistance
3. Balance (and posture)
4. Flexibility

On any given day, you can focus on just one type of activity or do a combination. The trick is to be consistent and stay active over time. It helps to be practical with what you choose to do. Consider picking just a few exercises each time you're active and regularly vary them. This can help you stay motivated while it provides optimal health benefits. We'll discuss each type of activity in more detail in the sections that follow.

AEROBIC ACTIVITIES: BUILDING ENDURANCE AND PHYSICAL FITNESS

By definition, an *aerobic activity* is any that is performed continuously for more than two minutes. We only define activities into types because the bodily systems they stress differ by type. Aerobic exercise helps to improve your endurance, fitness, blood flow, and heart health, along with increasing the mass of the muscle fibers at the lower end of the slowness spectrum and helping you maintain your body weight or lose fat.

Aerobic Exercise Types

Examples of aerobic activities include walking, swimming, rowing, cycling, dancing, using fitness machines, and more. Running and jogging are also aerobic in nature for most people (assuming they're not sprinting) but are high impact. Most people cannot continue to do these regularly over the age of 40 due to lower-limb joint pain and injuries. Fast walking is a good alternative as you get older.

Aerobic Intensity

How hard you work out doing aerobic exercise can vary widely (box 3.4). If you're just getting started with being more active,

68 • AGING WELL WITH DIABETES

> **Box 3.4**
> **What Is the Intensity of Your Aerobic Workouts?**
>
> - **Mild:** standing without support, slow walking (two miles per hour or less), some household chores (e.g., washing dishes), some gardening (weeding), using a buoyancy belt in a pool to walk or kick, playing shuffleboard, stationary cycling without resistance, and golfing using a cart
> - **Moderate:** walking briskly (level surface), swimming laps, cycling outdoors on a level surface, mowing, raking, hoeing, mopping or scrubbing floors, golfing while walking and carrying your clubs, tennis (doubles), volleyball, rowing, water aerobics or other aquatic classes, most chair exercises, and dancing
> - **Vigorous:** walking briskly (up an incline), climbing stairs, cycling up a hill, fast swimming, digging holes or shoveling, tennis (singles), cross-country skiing, downhill skiing, hiking, jogging or running, most sports (like soccer or basketball), and shoveling snow

you'll want to work up from the bottom of the intensity scale to avoid injuries or loss of motivation. Start with an easier pace, and slowly build up to doing more. At this point in your life, it's not a race to the finish (and if it were, it would be more like a marathon than a sprint), and you don't benefit by pushing too hard too soon. You're trying to stay active for the rest of your life, so you should pace yourself.

Younger to middle-aged adults should aim for an intensity that is moderate or vigorous for most planned workouts. When you're on the younger side, your goal is to exercise at a level that increases your breathing and heart rate and feels "somewhat hard" to "hard." To gain fitness, you don't need to work so hard that you can't talk to someone else, and your activity should not cause dizziness, chest pain, or excessive joint discomfort.

You can use your heart rate as a measure of your intensity as well, but your maximal pulse rate decreases over time and becomes less relevant. Dr. Colberg recommends subjective measures, such as how hard you feel like you're working overall with your entire body and your breathing, to monitor intensity instead of worrying about your heart rate. In fact, certain medications like beta-blockers can keep your heart rate artificially low during workouts in any case, as can diabetes-related complications that affect your central nervous system (such as *autonomic neuropathy*).

In addition to engaging in regular aerobic activities like walking, cycling, and swimming, it's helpful to add some faster intervals into any workout, such as walking faster for 10 to 60 seconds at a time during your normal walk or doing a hill profile on a cardio-training machine. Doing so will increase your fitness and improve insulin sensitivity for longer period of time. It's also possible to do high-intensity interval training (HIIT) at least once a week, but start out slowly and progress in steps to prevent injuries and demotivation— especially when you're older and intense activities create undue stress on aging joints that may not appreciate it. Furthermore, not all your workouts should be equally intense, and varying your aerobic activities lowers your risk of injury.

Aerobic Duration and Frequency

As far as the length of time you exercise, the recommended amount of aerobic activity for all adults is 150–300 minutes per week, which adds up to around 30–60 minutes per day on five days spread out over the week.[5,6] If you've been inactive, start out with an easy activity for 5–10 minutes daily, and increase the intensity and/or duration of your workouts over a few weeks to months. If it takes months to work up to the harder levels, don't get discouraged. Accomplish 15 or 20 minutes at a time and progress from there.

70 • AGING WELL WITH DIABETES

Studies have shown that for people with type 2 diabetes, exercising for shorter periods throughout the day that add up to the recommended amount can be as effective as (or even more so than) exercising all at once when it comes to blood glucose.[7] So fit it in whenever you can for as long as you can at a time. Frequent, short bouts of exercise can make the difference between "okay" blood glucose levels and more optimal ones.

Impact of Aerobic Activity on Blood Glucose

For most people with diabetes of any type, aerobic activity leads to a decline in blood glucose levels—and the longer you do it, the greater the decline over time unless you consume carbohydrates. Such aerobic activity will naturally lower elevated glucose levels, but be careful if you have a lot of insulin "on board" that you injected, pumped, or inhaled since any remaining insulin can cause your blood glucose to drop rapidly and too far during exercise. Exercising regularly will also allow you to require lower amounts of insulin, whether it's replacement insulin or what you produce on your own.[8]

A recent study on the "weekend warriors" who do a week's worth of exercise in only two days found that those individuals have a similarly low risk of heart disease and stroke as those who spread out their physical activity, but it didn't take diabetes into account.[9] For optimal blood glucose management, try not to let more than two days in a row elapse without doing some physical activity.[10] That's when the improvements in your insulin sensitivity start to wane. Since you're "only as good as your last aerobic workout" when it comes to insulin action, plan on an activity every day because you may occasionally miss a day or two per week for various reasons. It's fine to take at least one day a week off from planned activities to rest and recuperate a little, but try to do more unplanned activities on those days to keep your body moving.

Aerobic Activity Precautions and Considerations

To do aerobic and even resistance and other activities safely and effectively, consider doing the following:

- Including a warm-up period to ready your muscles for hard work. Do at least five minutes of a slower, easier activity first. After working harder for a time, repeat this easier activity as a cooldown period.
- Drinking fluids whenever activity is causing you to sweat, especially since the thirst center in your brain may not drive you to take in liquids as effectively as you get older.
- Checking with your doctor first if you're supposed to be limiting your fluids and refraining from drinking too much to avoid *water intoxication*. (Both chronic heart failure and kidney disease may require fluid restrictions.)
- Wearing layers of clothing you can remove during exercise, given that your body is less efficient at cooling itself down when you're older. Wear loose-fitting, light-colored clothing when exercising in the heat.
- Avoiding outside exercise during hotter weather, especially during the peak temperatures of the day. Stay out of direct sunlight as much as possible.
- Checking with your doctor if you experience excess pain in any joints (knees, hips, ankles, etc.) during activities or afterward. Some medications can help you stay more active without pain. Also, never overdo it or you may damage affected joints.
- Getting orthotics (a built-up shoe or inserts) to help decrease your hip or knee pain during activities if one of your legs is longer than the other.
- Choosing comfortable athletic shoes with gel insoles to wear during activities and pairing them with cotton-blend or athletic socks designed to keep your feet dry.

72 • AGING WELL WITH DIABETES

- Checking your feet daily for signs of redness, blisters, and ulcers and treating any potential problems early. If you can't easily see the soles of your feet, hold them over a mirror on the floor.
- Stopping and resting and talking to your doctor about your symptoms if you feel faint, dizzy, or nauseated or experience chest pain during activities.

If you're wheelchair-bound or unstable on your feet, you can still participate in aerobic activities. If your legs are able to move, you can do stationary cycling or many chair-dancing moves. It's also possible to use an upper-arm ergometer that allows you to cycle with your arms only. Chair dancing also involves arm movements that you can do while seated.

For safety's sake, everyone with health considerations or limitations should be aware of the common warning signs that may occur during aerobic exercise (table 3.1)

RESISTANCE TRAINING: BUILDING MUSCLE TO STAY STRONG

You may not be familiar with calling strength training "resistance training," but that's what it is. The whole goal of doing it is to recruit as many of your muscle fibers into action as possible, challenge them, and spur them to get stronger or limit their loss over time. As we mentioned, everyone starts losing muscle mass in their mid-20s (through a process called *sarcopenia*, or muscle wasting), and it accelerates as you enter your later decades (especially after the age of 60). You really need to keep your strength up in order to continue your normal activities, including caring for yourself and living independently (box 3.5).

STAND UP AND STRIDE AWAY • 73

Table 3.1. Symptoms After Exercise and How to Respond

Pain in your chest, left arm, or jaw	Stop and see if the pain resolves quickly. Contact your doctor about your symptoms. If pain persists, seek medical care or call 911.
Difficulty breathing or shortness of breath	Stop activity and see if your breathing returns to normal. If it doesn't, call your doctor (it may be a heart attack). If it's the result of exercise-induced asthma, use an inhaler. If your nose is dripping excessively into your nasal cavity, use a nasal steroid spray.
Dizziness	Stop and see if it persists. It may mean your blood pressure is too low. If it's from dehydration, drink fluids. If it still persists, consult your doctor as another condition may be causing it.
Muscle aches	Massage and heat the affected muscles. Lower your intensity or progress more slowly with activities to prevent aches.
Blisters on feet	Check your shoes for proper fit and cushioning, wear socks that keep your feet dry, and cover blisters with adhesive bandages. Contact a doctor or podiatrist if they persist or get worse.
Blood in urine	Stop activities and contact your doctor if it persists, especially if urine is dark in color (it could be from extreme muscle damage).
Diarrhea	Decrease the amount of exercise if it happens more than once. Consult your doctor if it persists.

The amount of strength you can gain from resistance training likely depends more on your training intensity than your age or health status, so almost everyone can benefit. Studies have shown that octogenarians (people in their 80s) can get stronger with training.[11] That's good to know since getting and staying stronger is crucial to preventing injuries, particularly those resulting from falling.

What's more, possessing more strength can help you lessen or prevent the muscle weakness that often results in pain, such as low

Box 3.5
Insight from Dr. Colberg

When I lecture to groups about the various types of activities that everyone with diabetes should be doing, a common question she gets is "If I only have time to fit in one physical activity, which one should I chose?" There's only one answer I ever give to that question, and it's "resistance training."

---

back pain. Any lower back discomfort can be debilitating and greatly affect your activities and your quality of life. It's often the result of sitting, which is an unnatural position for your back. Most of us sit way too much every day and with less than optimal posture. Lower-back-strengthening exercises can help you with your posture and get rid of that low back pain (or prevent you from ever feeling any).

You really need some resistance exercise on a regular basis to age well. Being inactive and living a sedentary lifestyle greatly accelerates your loss of muscle over time. Unfortunately, diabetes is also well documented as increasing rates of loss, especially when blood glucose levels are not well managed.[12] When you train aerobically, you probably aren't recruiting those fast twitch fibers we were talking about—even brisk walking doesn't bring all your muscle fibers into play. It really takes some fairly intense resistance exercises to do that. Even very small changes in muscle size can make a big difference in your strength and what you can accomplish, such as climbing stairs or even getting up off the toilet.

Women inherently have less upper-body strength than men, and having weak shoulder muscles is a common problem. In fact, by the time most women reach the age of 60, almost half can't lift 10 pounds, and more than 65% can't lift that amount once they hit their 70s. How are you going to carry groceries, lift a pot of water off the stove, or perform other chores around the house and yard or to take care of yourself if you're that weak? Resistance training may be your only salvation. Once you start training regularly, your strength can start to increase even after just a week (due to neural adaptations) without much change in your muscle size. After more weeks of training, your muscles may start to increase a little in size or appear more toned—and who doesn't want that?

Finally, your bones stay stronger when you regularly put normal stress on them, such as carrying your own body weight around when walking or jogging, doing resistance exercises with your upper body, or performing household chores. If you stay sedentary, your bones will lose minerals faster and thin out more quickly, and non–weight-bearing activities like swimming and cycling lack the same ability to build bone. Attempt to adequately stress your bones to keep your bone mineral density at high levels—at least two to three days per week.

Types of Resistance Exercise

You can increase your muscular strength in lots of different ways. Many people are now doing *body weight exercises*, which strengthen as a result of lifting your weight against gravity. For other strength training, you'll need weights or resistance of some sort, and there are many options for that without ever leaving your house or where you live.

For instance, you can use the hand and ankle weights sold in sporting-goods stores (starting with a small set of one-, two-, and five-pound dumbbells). Items around your house can work equally well, such as full water bottles, emptied milk jugs filled with sand or water, and socks filled with dried beans. Some people prefer to join a fitness center and use its equipment. Others buy resistance bands, which are sold at sporting-goods stores and online, usually for under $10. They're made from stretchy elastic, come in different colors for various amounts of resistance, and work for a number of arm, leg, shoulder, and torso exercises.

Which specific resistance exercises should you do? Check appendix A for some recommendations. At a minimum, for your arms and shoulders include double-arm raises (out to the side and up over your head), biceps curls (for the front of your upper arm), triceps extensions (working the back of your upper arm), and rowing exercises. For your legs, do exercises that bend and flex at the knees and hips, along with calf raises and side leg raises. If you work the muscles on one side of a joint (like the biceps), you should also exercise the opposite side (the triceps in this case). Abdominal work and low back exercises are also important to building core strength.

Of note, studies have shown that people with diabetes achieve better blood glucose management when they engage in more difficult resistance training that is supervised than when they do similar exercises at home on their own.[13] There may be many different reasons for this. If you need to kick-start your training program, you may want to begin in a supervised setting, both to increase your motivation and to learn the proper techniques for any unfamiliar exercises.

For basic mobility and self-care, you may simply want to try doing wall sits and/or sit-to-stand exercises. Many older people get heavier and weaker over time and start to have trouble with these basic maneuvers, making it harder for them to live well independently. To improve your ability, practice doing wall sits, which involve sitting against a wall for as long as you can with your hips and knees at 90-degree angles and your feet directly below your knees. This exercise will also help prevent knee pain and problems. Alternatively, you can do sit-to-stand exercises in which you sit on the edge of an armless chair and practice getting up without using your arms. (This is also often called the "getting up from the toilet" exercise.) You may also need to work on strengthening other areas of your lower body (box 3.6).

Resistance Intensity

Most studies have shown that moderate to intense levels of resistance training are required to see gains in your strength.[13,14] That's usually defined as at least 50% of the maximal amount you can lift one time (your so-called one-rep max) for moderate and closer to 75% or more for intense. Really, you should start out on the lower end and work your way up as much as you can without causing any injuries.

When you're older, you're much more likely to experience some joint limitations—be it from a former injury, arthritis or another degenerative disorder of the joints, or other reasons—and you may not be able to train as hard as you'd like. That's okay. Just do what you can and progress as you're able to get the most benefit.

Box 3.6
A Word about Working Your Ankle Muscles

The ankles are complex joints, and many problems arise when weak muscles allow them to roll too far in or out. Work on keeping your ankles strong to keep your balance, avoid falls, and prevent foot bone fractures and inflammation of the tendons around your ankles. Include a series of ankle-strengthening exercises in your weekly routine, and work on keeping ankle flexibility to avoid injuries and falls. Stretch the soles of your feet while you're at it.

Resistance Duration and Frequency

There is no set duration for the length of time you should do resistance exercises during each training session. Experts usually recommend that you try to fit in at least the following:

- 8–15 repetitions (or "reps" for short) per set
- 1–3 sets per exercise
- 8–10 or more different exercises that include muscle groups in the
  - upper body (arms, shoulders, neck, upper back),
  - lower body (hips, buttocks, legs, calves), and
  - core (abdomen and lower back).

We recommend that you start out at the higher end for the number of reps (12–15) and work your way down to doing more in the range of 8–12 at a harder resistance. Start out with 1–2 sets and work up to 3, or follow what Dr. Colberg does and do only 1–2 sets of any exercise and then a second exercise that works the same muscle group (for variety). You can obtain muscular strength and/or endurance gains from various combinations of sets and reps (box 3.7).

As for frequency, it's also recommended that all adults engage in at least two nonconsecutive days a week of resistance training but preferably three if you have diabetes.[5,6] Amazingly, studies have shown that training just one day a week can result in major strength gains in older adults, as can performing a single maximal lift once a week.[15,16] Of course, you'll probably gain more if you do more than that—but it's good to know that doing anything is helpful.

You should space out your resistance training so it doesn't occur on consecutive days because it usually takes muscles at least 48–72 hours to recover from damage incurred in the last training session. Of course, it depends on how hard you train (how many sets and reps at what resistance). Some people like to train more often and get around the every-other-day rule by working on different body

Box 3.7
Muscular Strength versus Muscular Endurance

You've heard people talk about "endurance" in the context of aerobic training, but it can also apply to resistance exercises. It is different from muscular "strength," though, and how you choose to train can have an impact on whether you're working on one more than the other.

Muscular strength: The maximal power that can be produced by a muscle. Think about how much weight or resistance you can lift at one time. That's how strong you are. To build strength, you have to focus on doing harder work with fewer repetitions.

Muscular endurance: How long a muscle can produce a certain amount of power over an extended period of time. For example, you may want to set a timer and do abdominal curls for a minute or until you get too tired to do any more. That works on endurance, not strength, because the intensity is lower and the duration is longer.

parts on subsequent days, such as emphasizing exercises for the upper back, shoulders, and arms one day and the lower body and abdominal muscles the next. If you're doing really light training, you can probably do it every day if you prefer without any issues with recovery time. That type of training is not going to increase your strength or lower your overall blood glucose as much, though, because of its lower intensity.[17]

Resistance Activity Precautions and Considerations

Resistance training is no good if you get injured or have to stop doing it. Here are some tips for staying safe and getting the most out of your resistance exercise sessions:

- If you're new to training, start out on the low side (for instance, using only one or two pounds of resistance or no weight other than moving your limbs).

- Gradually build up to using more weight; it's better to start out too low than too hard and injure your joints and muscles.
- Maintain control of your movements throughout each exercise at all times.
- Breathe out during the first part of the move and inhale slowly when you return to your starting position; never hold your breath because it raises your blood pressure.
- Wait two to three minutes between sets on an individual exercise; while you're waiting you can rest, stretch, or carry out a different exercise using another set of muscles.
- It's optimal to feel fatigued by the time you reach your target number of reps per set. If you can't reach 8, try a lighter weight; if you can do many more than 15, try a heavier one.
- It's possible to do variations of most resistance exercises either standing or seated, so you should be able to perform most of them from a wheelchair. Some can also be done lying down if you prefer.
- If you've had a hip or knee repair or replacement surgery, check with your doctor before doing heavier weights with the affected joints—and the same goes for shoulder replacements.
- Strengthening the muscles around replacement joints is crucial to long-term success with those new joints.
- Avoid bending your hips more than 90 degrees during any resistance exercises or jerking or thrusting weights into position; use smooth, steady movements.
- Don't lock your arm or leg joints in the straight position with a great deal of weight on them; doing so could cause injury.
- These exercises can cause a "burning" sensation in your muscles when you reach the end of each set, but they should never cause pain.

- Try to work through each joint's full range of motion when doing your exercises for optimal strength and flexibility.
- Mild muscle soreness lasting up to a few days and slight fatigue after training are normal, but severe soreness and sore joints are not; if your joints are sore, you may be overdoing it, so back off a little.

Impact of Resistance Activity on Blood Glucose

Resistance exercise has a variable impact on your blood glucose levels. When you do heavier lifting, it often causes a temporary increase in your levels, followed by a greater decline after a few hours. The increase is the result of a large release of glucose-raising hormones (like *adrenaline* and *glucagon*) and the relatively short duration of each activity when you lift more. A lighter resistance workout may have a minimal immediate impact on your glucose, or your levels may drop slightly. It also depends on the duration and not just the intensity of training, as well as the time of day you exercise. If resistance work does cause your glucose to rise, wait a few hours to see whether it decreases on its own before treating it since your body will be restoring the glycogen used during exercising.

BALANCE AND POSTURE: DOING EXERCISES TO HELP YOU STAY ON YOUR FEET

It's a sad fact, but balance ability gets worse with age, and it starts to decline around the age of 40. It is the result of neural (nerve) connections in the part of your brain that controls fine movement. The good news is that you can likely regain some of your balance ability with practice.

82 • AGING WELL WITH DIABETES

Let's test your balance right now to see how good it is (or isn't). Stand up and stand on one leg and then close your eyes. (Tip: Don't try this without holding on to something. We're trying to prove a point, not get you hurt.) If your balance is worse with your eyes closed, join the club—this is the case for everyone. Most of us rely more heavily on our sight to help us balance as we age, but even Dr. Colberg's college-aged students have trouble standing on one leg without vision to help them.

To balance effectively, your body relies on having strength in your hips and ankles, along with feedback provided from the nerves in your feet and signals sent back to your brain to determine your "position sense." The part of your brain called your *cerebellum* helps interpret the neural signals and keeps you upright and on your feet. Sometimes other conditions can interfere with your balance as well, including *autonomic neuropathy* (central nerve damage), vertigo, and other inner-ear issues.

Balance Exercises
Here's some more good news: All lower-body resistance exercises double as balance training. So when you're getting stronger, you're improving your balance at the same time. In addition, you can easily work on many other balance activities at home.

Simple Balance Practice
There's a really easy balance exercise that you can do anytime, anywhere. Just hold on to something with both hands and stand on one leg at a time. Once you feel stable, slowly release one hand. Do this two to three times a day on alternating feet. Within a couple of weeks or months, your balance will rapidly improve.

Use these more advanced balance techniques as your balance improves: (1) hold on with one fingertip; (2) don't hold on at all; and

(3) close your eyes (still without holding on). Have something nearby you can grab onto if needed, though.

You can really challenge yourself by moving your free leg in different directions (e.g., to the front, to the side, behind you) while standing on the other one. Or you can practice doing this while standing on an uneven surface, such as a cushion.

Other Balance Activities

The exercise form that originated in China called tai chi works well to improve balance. It's actually the basis for all the martial arts, which emphasize balance ability in various bodily positions (often with one leg raised). Other activities such as qigong and yoga also include balance elements. Studies in older adults have demonstrated that tai chi helps prevent falls and improves balance, muscular strength and endurance, and *proprioception* (defined as "perception or awareness of the position and movement of the body").

Anytime Balance and Proprioception Exercises

Here's a list of other exercises that you can work into your regular routine. All help with balance ability and have the potential to keep you from falling as easily. Do them as often as you like.

- **Stand on an uneven surface.** You can stand on cushions of various firmness or even pillows or a balance board. Then try standing on them with your legs alternating between being close together and far apart.
- **Stand in a different position or under various conditions.** Try standing with your head tilted to one side or the other or straight. Try assuming these positions with your eyes open and then closed. Other variations include keeping your hands at your sides or away from your body and talking or staying quiet while standing in these positions.

84 • AGING WELL WITH DIABETES

- **Walk heel-to-toe.** Walk in a narrow straight line by placing your heel right in front of the toes of your opposite foot with each step, allowing your heels and toes to just touch or come close to touching. Do this along a wall or handrail at first until it gets easier to maintain your balance. (This is also a sobriety test often used by traffic cops checking for buzzed drivers. As Dr. Colberg jokingly likes to say, "But Occifer, I'm not as think as you drunk I am. I can straight a walk line.")
- **Walk backward.** Do this along a wall or counter without looking back. Use your hand to steady yourself if needed.
- **Toe towel grab.** This involves bare feet and a towel on the floor. Practice grabbing the towel with the toes of one foot at a time, first while sitting and then while standing.

Posture and Your Balance Ability

Your posture affects how you balance your body since you use muscles to balance your upper body whenever you sit or stand. Our postures can worsen over time for many reasons, including slouching and spinal changes with aging. With age, our bodies tend to lean forward, which throws off our center of gravity. Frequent slouching can compress your spinal discs over time and cause neck and back pain, and poor posture increases your risk of becoming unstable on your feet and falling. Many people nowadays have bad posture from always looking down at a mobile phone or other device in their hands. Especially as you get older, good posture is very important to prevent pain and keep you on your feet.

Posture Exercise

To practice having better posture, try this exercise: Stand with your back against a wall with your heels out about two inches. Hold your chin down on your chest and then try to bring the back of your head to the wall with your chin still tucked in. (It's not as easy as it sounds. Most people over 50 have a lot of trouble doing it.)

FLEXIBILITY TRAINING: KEEPING YOUR JOINTS MOBILE

Like so many things, our joint flexibility decreases with time. Just compare the flexibility of a young child to yours today. Regardless of your age, it's inevitable that you're not as flexible now as you once were. Elevated blood glucose levels can also cause your joints to lose their range of motion more quickly. This is because excess glucose binds to joint structures like collagen, making them more brittle and less able to flex.

Why Flexibility Matters

Flexibility is important for helping you move and function well. You'll find that some joints have more movement than others. Having tight hamstring (back of thigh) muscles is very common and even has an impact on your ability to walk. They are likely also affecting your posture and balance, whether you realize it or not. Dr. Colberg found out after a series of overuse injuries affecting her foot and ankle that they were likely arising from inflexible soles of her feet. Working on stretching out the bottom of her feet (the *plantar* surface) for several years has allowed her to bend over and touch the floor better than ever before in her adult life and avoid further injuries.

Working on your flexibility is critical to lowering your risk of developing joint problems and joint injuries, not to mention avoiding falls. People with diabetes are more prone to joint-limiting conditions like "frozen shoulder," *tendinitis* (the inflammation of various tendons), trigger finger, carpal tunnel syndrome, tennis elbow, and others.[18-20] Stretching may not prevent all these problems, but it can

86 • AGING WELL WITH DIABETES

help limit their impact. So it's past time for some stretching exercises to keep the flexibility you have and add to it.

Flexibility Training and Exercises

Work on your flexibility at least two to three days per week.[6] It's helpful to stretch after any exercise training or at any other time you feel tight. It doesn't seem to matter whether you stretch before or after activities (or both), but it's always better to at least warm up your muscles with a light activity before you stretch.

Slowly lean into a stretch as far as you can without causing undue pain. It's recommended that you hold *static* stretches for 10–30 seconds and up to twice that long when you're older. If you're as impatient as Dr. Colberg and can't hold them that long, either repeat the stretch to add up to the full duration or try something like *dynamic* stretching (done through movement) rather than static stretching. Try to push a little further into the stretch as you repeat them or move through the range of motion.

Also include stretches for all your major muscle groups and stretch the muscles on all sides of your joints (like biceps/triceps or quadriceps/hamstrings). Some lower-body exercises include hip rotations, quadriceps stretches, ankle rotations, and calf stretches. For your upper body, include shoulder and neck rotations, upper-arm stretches (biceps and triceps), and wrist stretches. Some sample stretches are shown in appendix B.

Flexibility Activity Safety Considerations

- Always do a light warm-up before stretching for best results (like some easy walking or arm movements).
- Never stretch to the point of excessive or shooting pain. Go to the point of slight discomfort and hold stretches there or back off slightly.

- Never bounce during a stretch. It actually makes muscles tighten reflexively and limits movement. Make slow, steady movements instead.
- If you have had hip- or shoulder-replacement surgery, check with your doctor before engaging in stretching exercises or bending your replacement joints past a 90-degree angle.

ARE THERE ANY OTHER SAFETY CONCERNS WITH BECOMING ACTIVE?

If you've been inactive, can you just get up and start working out? How do you know if you need a checkup before you start exercising? If you're only going to do easy to moderate activities, such as brisk walking, most of the time you can start without seeing a physician.[6] Of course, if you have any troubling symptoms (like chest pain), you'd better rethink that. In any case, getting checked out before you start more intense activities can be a good idea. It also depends on how old you are, how active you've been recently, and your general health.

You don't want to start and then have to stop again immediately due to problems with your health caused by exercise. It's also possible to get sidelined by acute athletic injuries (like rolling your ankle) or develop an overuse injury (such as tennis elbow). You'll find out more about how to treat these injuries later in this step.

If your blood glucose is pretty well managed, you're already physically active, and you have no serious health complications, then feel free to stand up and be on your (active) way. Having to get a checkup if you're already working out regularly is unnecessary and can be a deterrent to becoming more active. If you have diabetes or prediabetes, though, regular medical checkups are always advisable.

Recommended Checkups for Exercise

If you're currently sedentary and starting an exercise program, you may benefit from having a checkup if any of the following apply:

- You plan on participating in vigorous activities, not just easy or moderate ones.
- You are over 40 years old (or over 30 if you meet any of the criteria that follow).
- You have had diabetes for more than 10 years.
- You have heart disease, a strong family history of heart disease, or high cholesterol.
- You have poor circulation in your feet or legs (or lower-leg pain while walking).
- You have diabetes-related eye disease, kidney disease, numbness, burning, tingling, or a loss of sensation in your feet and/or dizziness when going from sitting to standing.
- You haven't consistently managed your blood glucose levels well.
- You have joint pain, arthritis, or other chronic health problems that affect your working out.

Exercise Stress Testing

Most of the time you won't need to have what's called an "exercise stress test." That usually involves walking on a treadmill or using a stationary cycle for around 10 minutes and feeling like you're going up a big and never-ending hill (it's not much fun, in other words). It can sometimes be used to diagnose whether you have restrictions in the blood flow to your heart.

The American Diabetes Association recommends exercise stress testing only if you're over 40 and have diabetes or if you're over 30 and have had diabetes for 10 or more years, smoke cigarettes, have high blood pressure, have high cholesterol, or have eye or kidney problems directly related to diabetes.[6] If you have any concerns, check with your doctor at your next visit to discuss any measures that may be important for your health when exercising.

Recommendations for Specific Medical Conditions

You may need to make accommodations to exercise safely if you have certain medical issues, especially those such as exercise-induced *angina* (chest pain during activities only), vascular disease, chronic obstructive pulmonary disease (COPD), arthritis, and diabetes (table 3.2). Consult your doctor before starting or increasing the intensity of your exercise program.

MANAGING THE SIDE EFFECTS OF AGING AND BEING ACTIVE

While most of the side effects of being physically active are positive bodily changes, we would be remiss not to include some discussion of what to expect as you age and how to deal with any negative aspects. Those can include muscle soreness and injuries, to name a couple.

Remaining sedentary to avoid any possible downside to being active is clearly not the best thing for your health, but exercising excessively isn't either—there's a fine line between too little and too much activity. You have a greater risk of developing overuse and other athletic injuries as you age. So moderation in all things is advised when it comes to exercise as well. We'll talk a lot more in this section about adequate rest and recuperation time to avoid and manage overuse and other injuries related to being active.

Table 3.2. Exercising Safely with Common Health Problems

Chest pain	• Start new exercise training in a supervised setting, such as in a cardiac rehab program or physical therapy clinic. • If pain arises with harder exercise, alternate faster intervals with slower ones of one to two minutes. • If pain is severe (and being treated), take your medicine before exercising. • If cold weather makes your chest pain worse, exercise indoors.
Peripheral vascular disease	• Start with intermittent exercise (with interspersed rest) before moving on to continuous. • Be aware of the signs and symptoms of reduced blood flow to your legs and use pain as your guide. • Regular exercise should decrease calf pain. • Dress warmly for activities outside, and keep your hands and feet warm.
Chronic obstructive pulmonary disease (COPD)	• Do aerobic training (such as walking or stationary cycling) in the late morning or afternoon when your lungs feel more clear. • Exercise indoors in a moist, warm room when outside air quality is poor. • Start out doing one to five minutes of activity at a time and increase gradually.
Arthritis	• Consider doing water activities, cycling, and strength training to improve overall function. • Mild to moderate activities can improve joint pain over time, but avoid those that aggravate joints. Try alternative ones that are less irritating. • Avoid spinal flexion exercises if you have arthritis in your back, but include exercises that tone the abdomen and extend the spine.

Bodily Changes with Aging

Being active can prevent disability from premature aging due to chronic illnesses, but physiological aging is not entirely preventable.[21] Your running (and jogging and walking) endurance and maximal strength decrease with age due to combined changes in different bodily systems.

Your maximal heart rate decreases, your heart pumps out less blood, your muscle mass declines, your lung capacity gets lower, and your nerves conduct impulses more slowly. As mentioned earlier in this step, you're mainly losing the faster twitch muscle fibers that give you power and speed and, unfortunately, no matter how much you train, you can't get most of those back. For women, going through *menopause* (when monthly menstrual cycles stop) accelerates the loss of bone mass.

Bodily Changes Moderated by Activity

Being active on a regular basis has the capacity to prevent at least some of these declines. Working out can keep your accessory breathing muscles trained and stronger, which allows for deeper breaths. You'll lose fast twitch muscle at a slower rate if you do heavier resistance training (that recruits them into action). Although a person's maximum aerobic capacity typically declines about 1.5% per year, highly trained older athletes have a rate one-third of that (only half a percent per year), although it still declines some. Doing resistance training and weight-bearing activities stresses bones and slows the rate at which bone mass is lost.

Muscle Soreness Following Exercise

Whether starting a new activity or just overdoing a usual one, you may experience some soreness or stiffness for a day or two afterward—that's a normal response to the cellular damage you caused that needs repair. Don't let it discourage you from trying to be active. You'll start losing the training impact of any specific activity after taking just a week off, but you'll gain your level of fitness back faster than you did the first time you started the training.

Stretch out any tight muscles and joints after activities, and make sure to include gentle warm-up and cooldown exercises before and after every session. Forget "no pain, no gain." It's just not true. You never need to do anything to the point where it makes you really sore in order to benefit from it. Research suggests that muscle rebuilding (that is, *hypertrophy*) happens independent of any discernible damage to your muscles.

If you worked out so fiercely that your mobility around your joints is actually limited a day or two after a workout, you may be experiencing *delayed-onset muscle soreness*, which is caused by excessive overload to the muscles that leads to significant damage. Although uncomfortable, painful areas require no special treatment other than time, and the discomfort often feels better if you do some light exercise, stretch, gently massage the affected muscles, and take a hot bath or enjoy a stint in a hot tub or sauna. The pain usually peaks after 48–72 hours but may take 5 or more days to fully resolve. Luckily, your body should respond by building stress proteins into the repaired muscles, making it very hard to reach that level of soreness in the same muscles for six to eight weeks afterward, even if you overdo it again.

To avoid soreness and stiffness, try other recovery activities like using a foam roller to gently roll out sore muscles or taking a warm bath using Epsom salts. Heating pads can help with muscle soreness, and ice can help with inflammation. And if anything seems really painful, contact your doctor for further assistance.

Injury Management and Prevention

Injuries as a result of being active happen often enough that you need to know how to prevent and treat them. When you start exercising, you increase your risk of getting acutely injured or developing an overuse injury over time. The best medicine is prevention. If you can keep injuries from happening, you can avoid having to take time off from exercising and sidetracking your fitness.

Take a close look at the causes of injuries, which are the most common, and how to prevent and treat them for the best results. The judicious use of ibuprofen or another anti-inflammatory medication available without a prescription can help control the pain and inflammation associated with both acute and chronic injuries, but you may need to check with your doctor first. We'll talk about all of that in the next sections.

Dealing with Common Exercise-Related Injuries

Suffering with intense or lasting pain after exercise is not normal or expected. You can get an acute injury by using improper exercise techniques or through carelessness (e.g., dropping a dumbbell on your foot). If you ever feel a sharp, localized pain during or immediately after training, treat it with R.I.C.E. techniques (rest, ice, compression, and elevation; box 3.8). As soon as the injury improves, ease slowly back into your exercise routines and have a doctor examine anything that seems especially painful. You should also consider exploring other less painful exercise options.

Here are some of the more common acute exercise-related injuries that occur mainly in your shins, ankles, and feet:

Ankle sprain: A painful stretching or tearing of a ligament. *Inversion sprains* are common and occur when a foot twists inward, which excessively stretches or tears the outside ligaments.

Plantar fasciitis: Inflammation in the plantar fascia (the arch along the bottom of the foot). The main symptom is pain in your heel when standing or walking. Wearing shoes with poor arch support and very stiff soles and not stretching after exercise can cause this injury.

Heel spur: Abnormal bone growth on the heel that results from untreated or prolonged plantar fasciitis.

Shin splints: Occur during physical activity when too much force is placed on the shinbone and connective tissues that

> **Box 3.8**
> Treat Acute Athletic Injuries with R.I.C.E.
>
> - **Rest:** Stay off your feet as much as possible and use crutches if necessary.
> - **Ice:** Cover the area with a towel and apply a plastic bag full of ice to the injury for 10–20 minutes at a time several times a day for two to three days to help reduce swelling.
> - **Compression:** Use a pressure bandage (like an Ace or self-adhesive bandage wrap that can be wrapped around the affected area) to help reduce swelling.
> - **Elevation:** Elevate your lower extremity (like an injured ankle or foot) slightly higher than heart level to help reduce throbbing pain.

attach muscles to bone. You'll feel a sharp pain along your lower leg (shinbone) while exercising. This is caused by inflammation of the shinbone or stress fracture of the tibia or fibula (lower leg bones).

Achilles tendinitis: Inflammation and swelling of a heel tendon. The main symptoms are swelling, redness, pain, aching, and stiffness before, during, and after exercise, with pain that gets worse when walking uphill or climbing stairs. The usual causes are tight calf muscles, poor stretching habits, running on hard surfaces and hills, and wearing overused, worn-out shoes.

If you properly care for your injuries, they should start to improve within a week. If not, or if you have a single point of intense pain, you should see a doctor about it, preferably one with expertise in foot, ankle, and lower-leg problems as well as diabetes. Your doctor should be able to pinpoint the cause of discomfort with an X-ray, bone scan, or magnetic resonance imaging (MRI). Some people may need physical therapy or rehabilitation for persistent problems of the acute or overuse type.

Preventing and Managing Overuse Injuries

Getting more exercise is beneficial only up to a point, given that the incidence of activity-related injuries, such as inflamed tendons (*tendinitis*) and stress fractures in bones, rises dramatically when people engage in more than 60–90 minutes of moderate or hard exercise daily. This type of overuse injury is nagging and persistently uncomfortable rather than something with a more acute onset.

Overuse injuries occur following excessive movement of the same joints and muscles in a similar way over an extended period of weeks or months. If you develop an overuse injury, it's likely to be the result of excessive training or doing too much too soon. These injuries are more common when you have diabetes because elevated blood glucose can affect the health of your joints.

Here are some common causes of exercise-related injuries:

- *Footwear:* no arch support, shoes too tight or too big
- *Exercise errors:* too much exercise, progressing too quickly to higher exercise intensities, no stretching, no warm-up/cooldown
- *Faulty biomechanics:* high/flat arches, muscle tightness
- *Environment:* exercising on slick, muddy, wet, icy, or uneven surfaces

To prevent such injuries, progress slowly with your exercise program (particularly the intensity), choose safe activities to do, always warm up and cool down, and make sure you stretch regularly to stay more limber. For ongoing overuse problems, treat affected areas with R.I.C.E. combined with anti-inflammatory medications such as ibuprofen (Advil or Nuprin) or naproxen sodium (found in Aleve). Check with your doctor and make sure these meds are compatible with your other health issues; for some with kidney problems or other issues, they may not be. Avoid returning to normal activities until your symptoms resolve, or try alternate exercises that don't aggravate the healing injury.

To prevent the recurrence of an injury, once you resume normal activities work on strengthening the muscles around the affected area. Following a shoulder joint injury, for example, focus on doing resistance work using all sections of the deltoid muscle, as well as biceps, triceps, pectorals, and upper-back and neck muscles. Strengthening the muscles surrounding a joint takes some of the potential stress off the joint and can help you remain injury-free.

Preventing Other Athletic Injuries

You may also develop knee and lower-back injuries. To prevent acute knee injuries, it's best to avoid rapid changes in direction or landing from a jump, progress slowly in your exercise routine, choose safe activities, always warm up and cool down, and stretch the leg muscles on both sides of the joint. In addition, choose exercises that help strengthen the muscles around the knee, such as biking, the leg press, and chair squats.

As for preventing acute problems in the lower back, avoid heavy weight lifting, minimize making rapid changes in direction, choose safer activities, do not progress too quickly during your exercise routines, always warm up and cool down, and stretch the lower back and thigh muscles.

Chronic low-back pain is a common occurrence in adults in general and is often related to poor posture (see step 3 for posture exercises), excessive tightness, and bone thinning with aging that can lead to spinal degeneration and compression of the spinal nerves. Sometimes this can be corrected with surgery or steroid injections, but it can also be chronic and not easily treatable in much older individuals. Try to keep your core muscles (in your abdomen and lower back) as strong as possible, and do frequent stretching to relieve pain in the lower-back area.

Planned Rest to Prevent Injuries

Taking at least one day a week off to rest from planned activities allows the body time to recuperate and may prevent overuse injuries like tendinitis and stress fractures. It doesn't mean that you have to stop moving on "rest" days, though. You can keep moving all day long on your rest days to keep your blood glucose better managed. As discussed earlier in this step, it's also important to get enough sleep (seven to eight hours a night for most adults), which is when your body can repair, rebuild, and recover from your activities.

Potential Diabetes Impacts on Joints

Although everyone gets stiffer with age, diabetes accelerates the usual loss of flexibility, especially when your blood glucose runs high. Glucose "sticking" to joint surfaces makes people with diabetes more prone to overuse injuries like tendinitis and frozen shoulder. It may also take longer for your joint injuries to heal properly. The bones themselves can lose mass from longer exposure to elevated blood glucose levels, making fractures more common in people with any type of diabetes. The best method to prevent any of these issues is optimal blood glucose management (see step 1) and regular stretching to maintain motion around joints.

GETTING FITTER WITH CROSS-TRAINING

You will likely benefit from doing a variety of activities on a weekly basis, an approach known as *cross-training* (box 3.9). It's not about

AGING WELL WITH DIABETES

> **Box 3.9**
> **Start Cross-Training**
>
> - Choose a variety of enjoyable activities, and include all of them in an exercise program rather than just a single activity.
> - While you may really enjoy one particular activity, you can actually improve your ability in that activity by adding others that use similar areas of the body. For instance, if you like to walk, some cycling as well can make your legs stronger when you do walk.
> - Substitute these other activities every second or third day of exercise, or do different activities with every session, such as walking half the time and cycling the other half or doing resistance exercises.
> - Substitute as many different exercise activities as you desire.
> - Keep changing exercise activities to keep yourself challenged and motivated and to optimize your fitness.

doing trendy routines like CrossFit. It's really just about changing up your workouts so you can get more fit, avoid overuse injuries, and keep exercise fresh and fun. Each activity you do stresses your muscles and joints differently, which lowers the risk of injury. It adds variety to an exercise program when you include activities like walking, cycling, rowing, swimming, pool exercises, arm bike, weight training, yoga, tai chi, and more, and it gives you different options to choose from based on time constraints, weather, and other factors. It also allows you to rest some muscles without stopping exercising entirely. Alternating hard and easy days is also a great idea.

Cross-training helps you deal with injuries without losing all your prior conditioning while waiting for the injury to heal. If you have lower-leg pain, work out with your upper body and vice versa. Try alternating weight-bearing activities, such as walking, with non–weight-bearing ones (e.g., swimming and stationary cycling) to avoid hurting another part of your body while your injury improves.

Coming Back from Inactivity

If you're resuming exercise after a lapse or just starting being active for the first time, you'll likely need to begin at a lower intensity (lighter weights, less resistance, or a slower walking speed) to avoid burnout, muscle soreness, or injury. Even doing only 5–10 minutes at a time (instead of 30 or more) is fine to start.

If you really don't want to exercise, make a deal with yourself to do it for just a short time to get started (which is often the hardest part). Once you're actually up and moving, you may feel good enough to exceed the time you promised yourself you would spend. (This happens to Dr. Colberg every time she's tired and doesn't want to start working out. She feels better once she gets going and ends up doing the full workout anyway.) The key is to get yourself to begin exercising through any means possible. Walking is also excellent exercise, so if you're not the workout type, incorporate more walking into your daily routines.

You may also want to journal how exercising makes you feel physically. Chances are you'll have more energy and feel better overall once you get back to a better lifestyle. It's not a race to the finish—you're in this for the long term to enjoy a longer and healthier life. So even if you're just taking baby steps in the right direction, you will more likely reach your goals if you stick with it and pace yourself.

Exercise Recommendations for Older Adults

We talked about how much activity you should be doing, but we didn't really address the specific exercise guidelines that apply to older adults. Honestly, they're not much different than the guidelines for all adults, with and without diabetes, which also apply to older adults (aged 65 and older) as well. You should take your initial fitness level into account, however.

According to the federal recommendations from 2018, older adults should engage in moderate-intensity aerobic and muscle-strengthening activities, along with staying more active overall. Resistance training is particularly important to reverse the loss of muscle mass and prevent additional losses associated with aging and being inactive.[22] Flexibility training is also important, along with balance exercises, particularly for older adults at risk of falls. Breaking up sedentary time is associated with better physical function in older adults, and it may preserve your ability to take care of yourself and live independently.

Brisk walking, gardening, yard work, and housework are good examples of recommended moderate-intensity activities that help retain physical function, build strength, and expend calories. Even home-based interventions and tai chi programs for older adults may be effective in reducing any fear of falling and lead to greater physical activity participation.

When you can't do the recommended 150–300 minutes of moderate-intensity aerobic activity a week because of your chronic health conditions, simply try to be as physically active as possible, taking into account how your health status may affect your ability to exercise safely.

Having a disability that leaves you with limited mobility or in a wheelchair doesn't mean you can't be regularly active. Working just the upper body can increase mobility as you gain enhanced upper-body strength, endurance, and flexibility. Any type of activity can give you most of exercise's health benefits, even if you do it seated in a chair or wheelchair.

Injury Prevention by Activity

Older individuals are doing many different athletic feats, including climbing Mount Everest. But not everything is the same, physiologically speaking, for aging athletes. Older bodies are not as adept at regulating body temperatures, making people more prone to dehydration in hotter exercise conditions and to injuries in colder environments. They are also more likely to experience acute mountain sickness at high altitudes. It's possible to stay fit as you're aging, but getting older does lead to undeniable and inevitable declines in how your body works. It happens to everyone, no matter how healthy or active. World records for running and weight lifting are all lower in older athletes, even the most elite.

The first step in avoiding specific injuries is realizing that you're more prone to them and taking precautions to avoid them using targeted training and a modicum of common sense. Here are some tips for the more common activities.

Running and Jogging

Include a warm-up period to reduce your chance of injury. A loss of flexibility combined with worn-down joints (with less cushioning) means that your lower-extremity joints take more of a beating since they're bearing the stress rather than your muscles. Also, use pain as your guide if you have arthritis and take preventative actions like changing out your shoes regularly (to keep more cushioning available), increasing running mileage or intensity slowly, and making sure you have some rest days when you do other activities. Stretching regularly can help slow the loss of flexibility, but remember that you may have to find an alternative to running and jogging at some point in your life or run less far and/or less often.

Swimming

As an older swimmer, tearing your rotator cuff becomes more likely, especially if you keep stressing your shoulder joints as you did when you were younger. You may be able to reduce stress on your joints by avoiding the use of hand paddles (which can contribute to impingement syndromes), choosing not to use swim fins because they put more stress on your knees, and increasing swimming distances gradually.

Outdoor Cycling

Overtraining when you're an older cyclist can lead to compression or inflammatory syndromes involving nerve problems in the upper body, so you may have to cut back on your training to avoid these. Wearing padded gloves can help, along with not resting with too much weight on your hands during cycling and making sure your seat height is optimal to reduce stress on your knee joints. Also consider using a padded seat or padded cycling shorts to avoid inflaming your *urethra* (the duct through which you pee) and to prevent pressure sores between your legs when riding long distances.

Golfing, Tennis, and Pickleball

You're not safe even just golfing or playing tennis or pickleball. Common overuse injuries for these activities include shoulder problems; neck, lower-back, and wrist pain; and *epicondylitis* (golfer's or tennis elbow). It helps to warm up and stretch properly, but you'll also need to do strengthening exercises, particularly for your back muscles. Always focus on strengthening the muscles around any affected joints with targeted exercises to lessen some of the stress off the bone surfaces themselves. If you do get overuse injuries, taking time off from those activities and using anti-inflammatory pain medications can help.

Planning for Exercise Success

With diabetes, you'll benefit from keeping your physical activity regular. Try to plan ahead to ensure you fit some in nearly every day. If you take insulin, that's even more reason to stay consistent since you will have to manage your insulin levels during and following activities to avoid lows and highs. Planning ahead is a good approach to stay on track and be consistent.

Always listen to your body, though, so you know when to take a break from exercise. When you are active, warm up, cool down, and stretch to avoid injuries. Don't push yourself more than needed on any given day, and exercise at lighter intensities, at least to start. Work harder on some days and go easier on others if that helps keep you motivated and injury-free. As for diabetes management, keep a record of your activities and your glucose responses. Also note how you felt, what worked and what didn't, and what you want to change or try the next time to get the most out of staying active.

WHAT OTHER TYPES OF ACTIVITIES ARE HELPFUL?

We've gone through increasing daily movement, aerobic training, resistance exercises, balance and posture activities, and flexibility training—what more could there possibly be? At least a few more things, we think, can help your life quality.

Eye Exercises

Funnily enough, most people over the age of 50 find they need longer arms (to hold things away from their eyes to read them). Instead of getting reading glasses or bifocals, try some eye exercises to retain the strength and mobility of the eye muscles responsible for near-focus reading and distance vision. These include simple exercises like rotating the eyes in various directions and alternating between focusing on near and far and back and forth.

Pelvic-Floor (Kegel) Exercises

Here's another one for you to try that can help manage stress incontinence, which often happens to older women in particular when a small amount of urine leaks from your bladder when you cough, sneeze, laugh, bounce, jog, or jump (that is, a "stressor" occurs). This is more common in women who have gone through childbirth, but it can happen to anyone, including men. For more severe cases in women, specifically, topical estrogen cream, dissolving tablets, or ring insertion may be helpful.

A simple treatment consists of pelvic-muscle training called Kegel exercises. These pelvic-floor exercises may feel difficult at first, but they get easier as you do them. Allow up to eight weeks to fully see the effects. For best results, contract these muscles 50–100 times daily by doing as many repetitions as you can several times a day. And contract these same muscles before coughing or sneezing. As the strength and endurance of these muscles improve, it's just a bonus that you'll likely have greater sexual (orgasmic) pleasure as well.

- Everyone: During urination, try to stop and start your urine flow. Make sure you empty your bladder totally after you finish the exercises.
- Everyone: Tighten your anal muscles as if stopping gas from being released.
- Everyone: Imagine you're sitting on a marble and pretend you're lifting it up by tightening your pelvic muscles. Hold them contracted for as long as possible.
- Women only: Shift muscular tightness from your rear to your front vaginal area.
- Women only: Tighten your vaginal muscles around two fingers inserted into your vagina or a tampon inserted halfway.

Brain Exercises

Physical activity helps slow the rate of brain decline (both cognitive ability and memory) by ensuring adequate blood flow to the brain and stimulating various areas involved in voluntary movement. Try doing simple memory exercises (like memorizing lists and repeating them later) as well as regular physical activity to keep your brain in top form and lower your risk of dementia. Better yet, do memory exercises while exercising for the best results. For a longer discussion and more brain activities to practice, skip forward to step 7.

A FINAL WORD (OR TWO) ABOUT PHYSICAL ACTIVITY

A final word from Dr. Munshi: "All my fellows and medical students know that when I am rounding in the hospital with them, I never ride elevators. I always take stairs even if I am going 8 to 10 floors in the hospital. In fact, I would say that these 'exercise snacks' during day to day were very effective when I climbed up Mount Kilimanjaro in Tanzania recently, which is Africa's tallest mountain."

And here is another final word from Dr. Colberg: "I always practice what I preach when it comes to exercise. There are only a handful of days each year when I can say that I was truly inactive; all the rest I'm doing either a planned activity (like swimming, cycling, walking, and resistance training) or a lot of movement throughout the day. It just makes my diabetes management easier to be consistently active, and I know that regular exercise has been the majority of the reason that I'm still so healthy and vibrant after more than 57 years of living with type 1 diabetes."

You can enjoy so many health benefits by being more physically active. The rest of your life really depends on your adopting a more active lifestyle. It's never too late to start, and if you're beginning at the unfit end of the fitness spectrum, you can gain more from exercise than from anything else you do. Try to include some of all the activities listed here every week. Work up to at least 20–30 minutes of endurance activities on most days of the week to help lower your blood glucose, and take frequent activity breaks as you move more all day long. Do resistance training two to three nonconsecutive days a week. Practice simple balance and posture exercises. And stretch at least three times a week to maintain or improve your flexibility. It pays extremely well to be as active as possible as far as your health, longevity, and quality of life are concerned.

CHAPTER FOUR

Step 4: Boost Your Gut Health and Your Diet

Believe it or not, you're only as healthy as the bacteria in your gut. While it may not be a topic you care to spend much time thinking about, it's a fact that the type of bacteria residing in your intestinal track underlies almost all diseases associated with premature aging as well as preventable diseases, particularly if your gut becomes "leaky." Type 2 diabetes and insulin resistance are associated with having more of the wrong type of gut microbes. Both a leaky gut and inflammation may even contribute to the onset of type 1 diabetes and other autoimmune diseases.[1]

So how can you boost your gut health? Consider changing the composition of your gut bacteria through a variety of lifestyle changes, including better eating, physical activity, and stress reduction. Even though we'll spend most of this step talking about nutrition, it's really focused on your gut health. The two are completely connected, and your diet is critical to getting and keeping your gut bacteria healthy and happy (box 4.1).

108 • AGING WELL WITH DIABETES

Box 4.1

Step 4: Boost Your Gut Health and Your Diet

- What's old
  - Knowing that "junk food" is bad for you and trying (and often failing) to eat less of it
- What's new
  - Understanding that the health of your body and brain depend on the health of your gut (the friendly bacteria living there and its "leakiness")
- What you should be doing
  - Making food choices (and other lifestyle changes) that contribute to the health and integrity of your gut, which will also end up benefiting your overall health and blood glucose

---

HOW UNHEALTHY BACTERIA AND A LEAKY GUT MAY AFFECT YOUR HEALTH

Much of your overall health relies on your gut, otherwise known as your intestinal tract. A plethora of studies have begun to research the impact of food choices, physical activity, and other things on the bacteria that reside in your gastrointestinal system—usually called your gut *microbiome* or *microbiota*. These bacteria can affect your health in both good and bad ways. Your body is already host to over 100 trillion mostly benign bacteria that affect you in many ways, such as helping you digest the food that you eat, producing some vitamins (like vitamin K) in your gut, programming your immune system, preventing infections, and even influencing your mental health and behaviors. Your microbiome makes up an entire ecosystem that may influence the onset of certain metabolic, autoimmune, and aging-related disorders, including obesity, irritable bowel syndrome, some autoimmune conditions, asthma, depression, autism, and some cancers.[2] The type of bacteria that predominate in your gut can potentially affect whether you gain or lose weight, get diabetes, or develop other health-limiting conditions.

What also matters to your health is the integrity of the lining of your intestinal tract. It is normally semipermeable, which is necessary to let nutrients pass through the wall of your small intestine. It has a mucus lining that can absorb water and nutrients from the foods you eat and release them into your bloodstream, along with some vitamins made by good bacteria. It is supposed to act as a barrier to toxins, bacteria, proteins, and other substances, however. The problems arise when your intestines let too much through, meaning they are *hyperpermeable*—or in other words they "leak."

If you have a leaky gut, the normally tight junctions (formed with proteins like zonulin and occludin) allow these bacteria, toxins, undigested proteins from your diet, and other unhealthy agents to pass through.[3] The end result can be a heightened state of systemic inflammation that stimulates some of your normally dormant immune cells into action. A whole host of autoimmune diseases, including lupus, multiple sclerosis, and type 1 diabetes, are potentially associated with a leaky gut.[1,4]

It is still unclear whether chronic inflammation contributes to gut hyperpermeability and the resulting diseases or if the gut becomes permeable first, causing inflammation and disease onset. Some conditions such as irritable bowel syndrome can wear down the intestinal lining over time and lead to leaking. We do know that dietary choices, stress, and other lifestyle decisions may injure your gut lining and lead to intestinal permeability over time, so some of it may be within your control and preventable. For example, regular exercise appears to enhance the integrity of your intestinal wall, which would reduce your chances of getting a leaky gut.[5]

110 • AGING WELL WITH DIABETES

Among other testing methods, the protein *zonulin,* when measured in your stools or bloodstream, can serve as a marker for a leaky gut.[6] For a refresher on systemic inflammation and its impact on your health, return to step 2.

AIM TO EAT WITH YOUR (GUT) HEALTH IN MIND

In this section we're going to discuss how to choose foods that heal your body rather than harm it. We've already mentioned the impact that your diet can have on your gut microbiome. Just as eating more fiber can boost good bacteria, eating other foods allows some of the bad varieties to flourish. Aging also influences how well we absorb the vitamins, minerals, and other nutrients in our diet, with lesser amounts being bioavailable for the most part. It's not uncommon for older individuals to develop deficiencies in micronutrients like vitamin D and magnesium, and even the prescribed medications you take can have an impact on your levels.

Poor eating makes you more likely to fall ill or experience complications from illnesses. The reverse is also true: good eating can lower your risk for many preventable chronic diseases, lower inflammation, reduce insulin resistance, and boost overall health. You can also use food for medicinal purposes to help treat and manage any health conditions you may have or develop later in life. Of course, food cannot take the place of actual medications you may need, so consult your physician before eliminating any medications.

Many foods and diets qualify as healthier for you than the typical American fast-food diet (that's a low bar, honestly). One that always gets trotted out for people to try, especially in the diabetes world, is the Mediterranean diet—rich in olive oil, fish, and red wine—but it usually also involves trying to walk as much as people in Mediterranean countries have historically done. Still, a diet rich in the foods this diet is known for is a healthy upgrade from the more processed and refined foods of the American diet.

Simply cutting back on your intake of highly processed foods can help with blood glucose levels, and most people with diabetes can benefit from moderating their total carbohydrate intake without going completely "low carb."[7] Some studies have examined the benefits of vegan (plant-based) diets in diabetes and noted some benefits, although such diets tend to be higher in carbohydrates because most plant-based calories come from that macronutrient.

Here are some of our recommendations for dietary changes associated with successful aging:

- **Fiber:** Eat more fiber by choosing plant foods such as dried beans, whole-wheat bread, brown rice, bran, fruits, vegetables, and nuts and seeds.
- **Fat:** Choose healthier fats like olive oil and foods, including plant and animal sources, that are rich in omega-3 fatty acids.
- **Fatty fish:** Increase your intake of fatty fish—which is high in omega-3 fats—including salmon, mackerel, sardines, and herring, or take fish-oil supplements.
- **Veggies:** Eat at least three to five servings of vegetables daily, including fresh or frozen produce but not including the starchy ones (potatoes, corn, peas, etc.).
- **Fruit:** Consume two to three fruits daily, focusing on fresh or frozen whole fruit rather than juice and choosing those that are lower in carbohydrates, like berries, if blood glucose is a concern.
- **Protein:** Take in adequate amounts of protein in your diet, including getting all of the essential amino acids used to build muscle and maintain bodily health.

112 • AGING WELL WITH DIABETES

- **Fluids:** Drink plenty of fluids, particularly water, and supplement those with foods with higher water content like melons and many vegetables. Avoid sugary drinks like regular sodas, lemonade, and flavored iced teas.
- **Tea:** Drink steeped green or black tea to obtain more antioxidants (catechins) naturally in your diet (but instant tea has only minimal amounts).
- **Alcohol:** Only drink alcohol in moderation, which is no more than one alcoholic drink a day for women and two for men, and never in excess. A drink is defined as one 12-ounce beer, 5 ounces of wine, 1.5 ounces of 80-proof liquor, or 1 ounce of 100-proof liquor.
- **Spices:** Season your foods with mores spices, particularly those with known health benefits like turmeric, cinnamon, ginger, thyme, cumin, oregano, basil, sage, and curry.
- **Antioxidants and phytonutrients:** Consume a wide variety of colorful fruits and vegetables to gain the most antioxidants and phytonutrients to fight diseases.
- **Probiotics:** Eat yogurt with live bacterial cultures that act as *probiotics,* which are known to limit inflammation and improve health. Fermented foods like kimchi and kombucha also include live bacteria, and all are known to foster a better gut microbiome.
- **Prebiotics:** Choose foods with prebiotics such as oligosaccharides, a carbohydrate naturally found many plant foods, as well as fructans, inulin, and pectin.
- **Herbals:** Consider using some herbal supplements with proven effects, such as ginger for vertigo and alpha-lipoic acid (a strong antioxidant) for neuropathy.

Dr. Munshi tells her patients—all of whom are 70 years and older—that changing their diet can be particularly difficult after so many years of certain eating habits, a lack of access to healthier choices, and other obstacles. So don't expect miracles and don't try to make too many changes too quickly to avoid getting tired of it and falling back on your old habits. Take one step at a time, and be cognizant of what you're putting in your body.

GET PLENTY OF FIBER IN YOUR DIET

Having a healthy gut microbiome may help to prevent a leaky gut. Before we get more into everything you can eat to improve the numbers of "good" bacteria in your gut, let's talk about fiber (box 4.2). It's so important that it deserves to be called out on its own. One of the most important elements of a healthful diet is naturally occurring fiber, which is abundant in plant-based foods like fruits, vegetables, whole grains and cereals, legumes, and nuts. Good bacteria in your gut thrive on fiber, and keeping those particular bacteria happy eating fiber can reduce your body's systemic inflammation.[8] Think about eating as much fiber as possible to keep your health optimized.

The American diet on the whole is seriously lacking in dietary fiber. Most processed foods contain very little since milling whole wheat into white flour removes all of the bran on the outside, which

---

Box 4.2
Insight from Dr. Munshi

Your gut's health is not only important for diabetes but is also critical as you age. A good diet and good gut health grants an overall feeling of well-being to people living well into their later years. It's crucial to choose foods and activities that promote growth of the good bacteria in your system, which may mean consuming more natural fiber, prebiotics, and probiotics.

114 • AGING WELL WITH DIABETES

is the part with the fiber. Some food manufacturers add fiber back in, but it's seldom as good as what is in foods naturally, and it's rarely in the same quantity. Even bumping up your fiber intake with that from a drugstore (like Metamucil) is never as good as getting it from the natural source.

REAPING THE HEALTH BENEFITS OF FIBER

What does fiber do for your gut health and your overall well-being? We know that it can bind onto cholesterol and pull it out of your body through your intestinal tract. It also increases the bulk of your bowel movements—which, admittedly, some people complain about, especially after eating legumes and beans—and keeps you more regular and less likely to be constipated. It's not uncommon to suffer from constipation more easily as you age, particularly if you are dehydrated at all, which can happen anytime your blood glucose levels are elevated enough to make you pee out extra fluids. Another reason to eat more fiber is to help prevent diseases that can cause premature death, such as heart disease, colorectal cancer, obesity, high blood pressure, and diabetes.

Finding Dietary Fiber in Plants

If you go looking for fiber in meat or dairy products, you're going to be sorely disappointed. Natural fiber is mostly found in plant foods—and the closer to nature the better. Manufacturers are required to list the grams of fiber per serving on food labels, but most of the best sources of fiber don't come with food labels because you find them in their natural state in the produce section of your grocery store (box 4.3).

Box 4.3
Where to Look for Fiber in Your Food

- Legumes (beans and peas)
  - Black, garbanzo (chickpeas), kidney, navy, lima, and pinto beans, along with lentils and soybeans
- Vegetables
  - Almost all veggies but especially green, snap, and pole beans; kale, collard, and turnip greens; Swiss chard, spinach, broccoli, Brussels sprouts, carrots, sweet potatoes, and fresh corn
- Fruits
  - Whole fruits that include skins but not peels for all berries (blueberries, strawberries, raspberries, blackberries), apples, oranges, pears, plums, cherries, kiwi, and guava
  - Dried fruits, such as apricots, cranberries, raisins, prunes, and others, but these may affect blood glucose more because they are carbohydrate dense and could have added sugars
- Whole grains
  - Oats, brown rice, whole-wheat or whole-grain breads and pastas, oat and wheat bran, rye, buckwheat, milled flaxseed, high-bran cereals, soy flour, cornmeal, and popcorn
- Nuts and seeds
  - Almonds, cashews, walnuts, pecans, pistachios, Brazil nuts, sunflower seeds, and peanuts (technically a legume)

Of course, since low-carbohydrate foods are still trendy, many manufacturers have found ways to bump up the fiber content of things like low-carb tortilla shells and protein bars. Fiber is either not digested or minimally digested in your gut, but the good bacteria residing there help to break it down. Mostly, it ends up increasing the amount of fecal matter you excrete (which is generally beneficial and lowers your colorectal cancer risk) and may also bind onto cholesterol and help excrete it from your body through your feces as well. Manufacturers also regularly add fiber to products like pasta, cereals, and breads. On food labels, "total fiber" doesn't differentiate between naturally occurring and added fiber but includes all sources.

Getting Enough Daily Fiber

The recommended intake of daily fiber varies with your age, and older individuals may need less because it's based on calorie intake— and you will likely need fewer baseline calories later in life. It also varies with biological sex, again because women usually need and consume fewer daily calories than men (table 4.1).

Unless you're really working hard at it, it's likely you're not currently getting enough fiber in your diet. Eating as much fiber as possible will benefit the health of most people, young or old, and is recommended. Think of it this way: Paleo diets are touted by many following trendy dietary patterns to manage chronic diseases, but despite the impression that Paleo eating involves mainly meat, it's estimated that by eating roots and berries early humans consumed at least 100 grams of fiber daily. Compare this with the US Department of Agriculture's recommended intake levels and you'll see that we're a long way from that.

Dr. Colberg has taught nutrition related to sports, fitness, and health to thousands of college and graduate students over the years,

Table 4.1. USDA Recommended Daily Fiber Intake for Adults

Age	Men	Women
19–50 years	38 grams	25 grams
Over 50 years	30 grams	21 grams

and she always challenges them to take in 50 grams of fiber naturally through food choices every day. One potential downside of eating that much fiber—other than being extremely regular and having larger volumes of feces to excrete—is its potential to interfere with the natural absorption of calcium and iron in your diet. If you do consume as much fiber as recommended (or more), drink plenty of fluids to stay hydrated and make sure you're getting enough of those minerals in particular.

Another downside of switching over to eating more fiber is the potential for increased intestinal gas—yes, more farting. One way to prevent this is to increase the fiber in your diet in gradual increments so that your body has time to get used to it. Don't add all the fiber-rich foods at once. Add just one or two servings a day to your regular diet for a week. Maybe eat whole-wheat bread on your sandwich at lunch or enjoy a salad at dinner. Give your body some time to adjust and add more servings the following week. Keep doing this until you reach your target amount.

Sometimes even with your best effort, you may be unable to get enough fiber through your diet alone. In those cases it's okay to take an over-the-counter fiber supplement like Metamucil, Benefiber, Gogo fiber gummies, or other varieties. This is also true for anyone with chronic constipation who may need additional fiber supplements.

FOCUS ON OTHER HEALTHY COMPOUNDS IN FOODS

Next, let's talk about how to get the most out of your food choices (besides eating more fiber). Foods that qualify as prebiotics and probiotics play a special role in gut health, and some of the compounds found in plants have other healing powers.

Eating More Prebiotics and Probiotics

Both prebiotics and probiotics are known to enhance health, particularly gut health. *Prebiotics*, specifically inulin and fructooligosaccharides, cannot be digested by the human body. Instead they stay in the bowel and help the good bacteria thrive, supporting a healthy digestion and gut microbiome. Foods with prebiotics include onions, garlic, apples, oatmeal, asparagus, ground flaxseed, and seaweed, among others.

Probiotics are live microorganisms that when administered in adequate amounts confer a health benefit on the host. Foods with these include sauerkraut, yogurt, natto, green olives, tempeh, kombucha, kimchi, apple cider vinegar, pickles, kefir, and miso. A recent study suggested that such food sources have the greatest ability to lower blood glucose levels and insulin resistance in people with type 2 diabetes.[9]

Accessing Other Healing Compounds in Plants

We've discussed how important fiber and healthier food choices can be for your health, and let's specifically address the disease-fighting power of certain compounds found exclusively in plants: phytonutrients and antioxidants. Certain antioxidants (like glutathione) have been shown to be particularly beneficial when you have diabetes. Aim to eat a wide variety of colorful fruits and vegetables—at least five servings a day—not only to boost your fiber intake but also to lower inflammation and promote health.

Phytonutrients

Plants contain special compounds called *phytochemicals*, or as we prefer to call them, *phytonutrients*. They have various proven health benefits. For instance, the lutein found in cooked tomato products (sauce, paste, etc.) has been found to reduce the risk of prostate cancer, and compounds in onions (mainly onionin A, cysteine sulfoxides, quercetin, and quercetin glucosides) can lower your risk of a heart attack or stroke. Some phytonutrients can also fight the damaging effects of sun exposure. While some of these compounds have been made into pills and bottled up, phytonutrients and antioxidants in natural foods work together synergistically, and it's always better to consume them naturally if you can.

Antioxidants

Many phytonutrients have antioxidant qualities. This is important because your body is constantly creating unstable molecules called *oxidants*, or free radicals. To stabilize, oxidants "borrow" electrons from nearby molecules but can damage your cellular proteins and genes (DNA and RNA) in the process, making those cells more likely to develop inflammation and even cancer. The phytonutrients that act as antioxidants help prevent such damage and premature aging. You can find antioxidants such as *flavonoids* in abundance in cocoa beans, dark chocolate, black and green teas, coffee, cranberries, peanuts and other legumes, strawberries, apples, blueberries, kiwi, cherries, avocados, sweet potatoes, winter squash, purple cabbage, eggplant, and dark-green leafy veggies . . . and the list goes on (box 4.4).

Eating a variety of colorful produce is your best bet. Aim to consume darker-colored foods because they're packed with phytonutrients. The dark outer coatings contain more antioxidants to protect the plants themselves against sun damage. For instance, beans are high in flavonoids, with black beans highest and white beans lowest (and red, brown, and yellow in between). Red and purple grapes have more disease-fighting power than green ones.

When you have diabetes, getting more of the highly colored foods—assuming the coloring is natural—may have additional health benefits. Anthocyanin, which adds a red color to tart cherries,

Box 4.4
Add More Natural Color to Your Diet

If most of the foods you eat are "white" ones like white bread, rice, potatoes, sugar, and iceberg lettuce, you need to up your color game when it comes to your eating. Phytonutrients in your produce vary with the pigment and in their ability to fight certain diseases. For optimal health, you should choose plant-based foods from at least four color groups every day. An example of a food and its disease-fighting power for each group follows:

Green: sulforaphane in broccoli helps prevent cancer.
Red: lycopene in tomatoes may help prevent prostate cancer in men.
Orange-yellow: carotenoids in carrots and sweet potatoes fight heart disease.
Blue-purple: polyphenols in blueberries are a powerful antioxidant.

---

red grapes, strawberries, and more, may have a positive impact on beta cells' insulin production. Try to eat your veggies raw, lightly steamed, baked, or microwaved instead of boiled, unless you want to drink the water they were boiled in to get all the nutrients that ended up there. One exception is tomatoes, which release more lutein when cooked.

Glutathione and Alpha-Lipoic Acid

Two of your body's antioxidants in particular, *glutathione* and *alpha-lipoic acid* (ALA), are critical to your long-term health, especially when you have diabetes. Glutathione is the main antioxidant enzyme found in all your cells and, along with ALA, is the most important antioxidant in your body because it protects against DNA damage via oxidation. Diabetes may increase your need for glutathione and ALA by depleting the former during blood glucose elevations. Your body can synthesize both of these from amino acids found in protein, but it helps to get more through foods like asparagus, avocados, spinach, strawberries, peaches, melons, and citrus fruits if you're not making enough.

ALA boosts glutathione levels by helping your cells absorb a critical amino acid needed for its synthesis. By itself, ALA can lower your risk for stroke, heart attacks, peripheral nerve damage, cataracts, memory loss, cancer, and premature aging. You can find ALA in abundance in spinach (raw or cooked) and in lesser amounts in broccoli, tomatoes, potatoes, peas, and Brussels sprouts. Spinach is especially touted for its ability to fight diabetes-related cataracts and macular degeneration, which is the leading cause of blindness in all adults.

Cataracts involve glutathione deficiencies in the lens of your eye, and ALA, vitamins E and C (both with antioxidant qualities), and selenium (an antioxidant mineral) can increase your levels of glutathione and better protect your eyes and other tissues. ALA supplements have been used to normalize kidney function and regenerate peripheral nerve fibers, and they're also used to treat painful neuropathy in the feet and hands and improve autonomic (central nervous system) neuropathy. Most people can safely take 600 milligrams (mg) once or twice daily for relief of symptoms.

KNOW YOUR FATS TO PICK HEALTHIER OPTIONS

Much has been published about the unhealthiness of certain fats and the health benefits of others. While that is generally true, too many oversimplifications of fats into various categories have definitely muddied the waters. Here's your primer on what to know about the fats you choose to eat.

Consuming Essential Omega-3 and Omega-6 Fats

Certain types of fats can't be made in your body and have to come from dietary sources (making them *essential fats*). One of these, omega-3 fatty acids, is found in cold-water fish and considered heart-healthy. The Japanese, some of the longest-living people in the world, often consume as many as 7% of their daily calories in the form of fat-rich fish (while Americans get less than 1%). Recent studies have shown that a diet higher in alpha-linolenic acid—which is the main omega-3 fat—lowers your risk of dying from anything, especially heart disease.[10] Omega-3s are also associated with better brain function, an improved ability to fight off illness, less cancer, a lower risk of heart attacks, and a lower chance of developing Alzheimer's disease. Almost all of these benefits are linked to a greater intake of the omega-3 fatty acids themselves.

Fish with plenty of omega-3 fats are best, as found in salmon, mackerel, and herring (table 4.2), and fish oil or omega-3 supplements can contain up to 1.8 grams as well. Getting too much mercury by eating longer-living fish has the potential to cause some health problems, however, so vary what types you eat, and limit your intake of predator fish like shark, swordfish, and mackerel. Also, choose the light or skipjack varieties of canned or fresh tuna, and eat the albacore, yellowfin, and bigeye tuna more sparingly.

Where else can you get more of the essential fats you need? Heart-healthy omega-3 fats can also be found in whole grains, seeds and nuts, leafy green vegetables, and certain oils like flaxseed, canola, and olive. Vegetables and some nuts and seeds (particularly walnuts and chia seeds) contain large amounts of omega-3s. Flaxseed oil contains 8.5 grams of omega-3 fat per tablespoon, while flaxseed or linseed contains 2.2 grams. Also look for it in canola oil (1.3 grams per tablespoon), soybean oil (0.9 grams), walnuts (0.7 grams), and olive oil (0.1 grams). Dr. Colberg knew an older man with type 1

Table 4.2. Omega-3 Fat and Mercury in Fatty Fish

	Omega-3 fat (grams per 3.5 ounces)	Mercury (parts per million)
Anchovy	1.40	0.04
Bluefish	1.20	0.34
Flounder or sole	0.43	0.05
Halibut	0.40–1.0	0.26
Herring	1.71–1.81	0.04
King mackerel	0.34–2.20	**0.73**
Mullet	0.60–1.10	0.05
Pollock	0.46	0.06
Sablefish	1.40	0.22
Salmon	0.68–1.83	0.01
Sardine	0.98–1.70	0.01
Shark	0.50–0.90	**0.99**
Sturgeon (Atlantic)	1.40	0.09
Swordfish	0.20–0.70	**0.98**
Tilefish (Atlantic)	0.80	0.15
Tilefish (Gulf of Mexico)	0.80	**1.45**
Trout (freshwater)	0.84–1.60	0.07
Tuna (all species)	0.24–1.60	0.38
Tuna (bigeye)	0.24–1.60	0.64

Notes: Only fish higher in omega-3s are included. Actual content varies by fish location. The FDA upper limit for mercury is 1.0 parts per million.

diabetes who put a tablespoon of milled flaxseed (also high in probiotics) into his cereal every morning—and he lived to be over 102 years old and participated in the Senior Olympics well into his late 90s. Coincidence? It's hard to say but worth considering. If nothing else, it certainly can't hurt to try it.

Omega-6 fats are also considered essential, and you can find these naturally in plant foods like nuts (walnuts, pine nuts, and Brazil nuts), seeds, and plant oils such as sunflower, safflower, and corn. Early humans consumed more of a balance of omega-3s and omega-6s, but today people consume many more of the latter and fewer of the former (about 10 to 1) due to the widespread use of vegetable oils. It's better to try to balance out your intake of the two types.

When it comes to diabetes management, the fat in your foods has less of a direct impact on your blood glucose than carbohydrates or protein because fat is digested slowly over three to six hours. Eating a lot of fat can make you more insulin resistant in some cases, but it really depends on what other calorie sources you replace it with. You shouldn't cut back on the fats in your diet excessively since low-fat diets can lead your liver to make and release more cholesterol, especially if you eat too many highly processed carbohydrates in their place.

An "anti–fat in foods" movement back in the 1990s resulted in manufacturers creating fake fats and fat substitutes (most of which gave people the runs). Others simply took fat out of foods to make them low fat, but they had to replace the fat with something, often refined carbohydrates or sugar. It wasn't a great time for people with diabetes concerned about managing their blood glucose levels. Dr. Colberg can remember people with diabetes eating low-fat cookies to treat low blood glucose events because those cookies were so high in sugar. Eating low-fat cookies is more likely to cause your cholesterol levels to rise than any type of fat.

Since we believe that moderation in eating works best, aim to take in about 30% of your dietary calories in the form of healthier fats. Also, despite what you've been told about cholesterol in foods, how much of it you eat has very little effect on your blood cholesterol levels and types. Your body uses cholesterol—which is a fatlike substance—to form cells and hormones, and your liver will create more cholesterol if you need it. In fact, plants do not contain any cholesterol. It's only found in animal meats and products, such as beef, poultry, pork, shellfish, eggs, and dairy. In the paradox of all times, eating eggs (with yolks rich in cholesterol) apparently will not raise your blood cholesterol, but eating refined carbohydrates (containing no

> **Box 4.5**
> **The Health Benefits of (Dark) Chocolate and Cacao**
>
> Yes, some types of chocolate are considered "healthy," and usually, the darker, the better. Despite containing some saturated fats and sugar, dark chocolate and cocoa can prevent oxidation and clogging of arteries because of their many flavonol compounds, which act like a low-dose aspirin and increase blood flow while lowering the risk of cardiovascular disease. Hot cocoa made with two tablespoons of pure cocoa powder is one of the best sources, containing two to five times the flavones of red wine, green tea, and black tea.
>
> Another option is brewed cacao, which is roasted, ground, and brewed like coffee. It has a rich, chocolatey flavor and is considered a superfood. It's similar to hot cocoa but without the extra processing. Most people think it's more like drinking coffee or tea.
>
> Given that Dr. Colberg is a recovering (dark) chocoholic, she would much rather eat dark chocolate (in moderation) or drink hot cocoa for heart health. If you make it sugar-free or choose brewed cacao as an alternative, it will benefit your blood glucose levels as well and with fewer potential negative side effects than taking a blood-thinning aspirin a day to prevent stroke.

cholesterol) certainly can. Dark chocolate and cacao can also be healthy (box 4.5).

Limiting Saturated and Highly Processed Fats

While you may love eating meat, the jury is out on its healthiness for you. Myriad research studies over the years have linked heart disease and certain types of cancer with a greater intake of red meat and pork (mammals) in particular. Early man didn't suffer from heart disease, but he also didn't live as long or consume any meat that he didn't have to chase down himself. Modern beef and pork sources are designed to be very fat-rich instead of lean like they used to be. Even poultry, and some farm-raised fish, is raised to increase its total fat content. Americans also consume a lot of high-fat cheeses and other dairy products (like ice cream).

Much of the fat from animal sources is more highly *saturated*, which makes it harder for your body to metabolize and leads to greater inflammation. The recommendations for years have been to decrease one's intake of saturated fats (which are typically solid at room temperature) and increase one's intake of *monounsaturated* and *polyunsaturated* fats like those found in olive oil, avocados, nuts and seeds, and other mainly plant sources. It's worth eating more plant-based fats and not just animal-based ones. Even tropical oils like coconut, if minimally processed, are now considered healthier options even though most of their fats are saturated.

What may damage your health even more is eating highly processed meats (like lunch meats, bacon, and sausage) and *trans fats*, which are created artificially when oils are altered to change their texture and extend their shelf life.[11] While their quantity now must be listed on food labels, they're often disguised as hydrogenated or partially hydrogenated oils. Research has shown that they can make you more insulin resistant, not to mention increase your heart disease risk.[12] Trans fats are often added to many varieties of crackers, cookies, baked goods, and more and are also found on ingredient lists as monodiglycerides, diglycerides, stearate, palmitate, lard, and vegetable shortening. Some trans fats occur naturally in cheese and other foods in limited quantities.

Fast food doesn't usually come with easy-to-find ingredient labels or nutrition facts, but you should know that eating it can make your blood flow sluggish and your insulin less effective for hours after a meal. Additionally, your blood cholesterol levels may decrease if you eat fewer highly processed and trans fats. It's just better to stick with foods closer to their natural state where your health is concerned.

MAINTAIN YOUR STRENGTH WITH PROTEIN

Muscles and other proteins in your body are made out of building blocks called *amino acids*. Your body makes some of them, but about half of the 20 amino acids are essential to have in your diet, just like some types of fat. With aging, taking in enough of these protein building blocks becomes even more important than when you were a younger adult. As you age, muscles don't repair as quickly or easily. You want to be able to form, maintain, and repair all the protein structures in your body, including not only muscles but also immune cells, hormones, enzymes, and much more. Your daily intake should be closer to 1.1 grams of protein per kilogram of body weight (1 kilogram equals 2.2 pounds), up from 0.8 grams when you were younger. Exercising a lot usually bumps your needs up to 1.1–1.6 grams per kilogram, depending on the type and duration of your activities.

High-protein diets have been a recent fad, and that's not necessarily a bad thing. If you eat as much as 30%–40% percent of your daily calories as protein, with a lower intake of carbohydrates and fats, you may find it easier to manage your blood glucose and lose weight. Protein has a high satiety factor, meaning that it keeps you feeling full longer. You don't want to have a high intake of protein from processed meats, though, as that can increase inflammation. Choose high-quality sources of protein like lean meats, soy products, legumes, fish, and nuts and seeds. Soy protein has even been shown to lower heart disease risk in adults with type 2 diabetes and keep their kidney disease from worsening as it lowers blood glucose, blood fats, and C-reactive protein (an indicator of inflammation).

As for protein supplements, a plethora of studies have focused on the impact of taking supplemental amino acids (the essential ones like leucine, found in whey protein from cow's milk) or even creatine to try to increase muscle mass in combination with resistance training.[13] While certain supplements may help weight lifters and power athletes when taken strategically, getting adequate amounts of amino acids through your diet is generally better because they're more balanced and "complete." That means they provide all the amino acids in the right combinations and quantities. Certain plant sources lack specific essential amino acids but can be combined with other foods to get complete protein, such as pairing beans and rice. In some cases, creatine supplements may help improve muscle mass and strength in older individuals.

HANDLE YOUR CARBOHYDRATES

Since consuming carbohydrates has the most immediate impact on your blood glucose, you may wonder why we would put this topic *after* our discussion of fiber, phytonutrients, fat, protein, and other items. The reason is because the only essential carbohydrate in your diet is fiber, and we started our entire discussion talking about that. The rest of the carbohydrates are mainly relevant due to their ability to be used as fuels during exercise and their impact on your blood glucose levels. If your body needs more glucose, it can either be made by your liver from precursors found in your body (like lactate, pyruvate, alanine, and glycerol), or your liver can release stored glucose. Hence, it's not essential in your diet.

The latest dietary recommendations for *macronutrient* (carbohydrate, protein, and fat) intake suggest you get your daily calories as follows:

- **Carbohydrate:** 45%–65% (four calories per gram)
- **Fat:** 20%–35% (nine calories per gram)
- **Protein:** 10%–35% (four calories per gram)

You can easily go as low as 40% of your calories coming from carbohydrates (or even lower) when you have diabetes, and it may make your blood glucose management a little easier, as can picking those that are digested more slowly. Keep in mind that the calories in fat add up much more quickly since each gram of fat has over double the calorie content of carbohydrate or protein sources.

You don't have to go extremely "low carb" with your eating, but some people with diabetes of all types choose to cut out almost all carbohydrates except for those in certain veggies and nuts and seeds. You really have to enjoy animal meats and products to cut out so many carbohydrates since all plant foods are higher in carbohydrates than protein or fat, with the exception of olives, avocados, coconut, nuts, seeds, and some legumes like peanuts. It's hard to eat like a *vegan* (that is, no animal meats or products) and also follow a low-carb diet.

Honestly, the types of carbohydrates you eat likely matter more than the total amount, although both play a role in your resulting diabetes management. Some are slowly digested and absorbed and raise blood glucose levels slowly or minimally after eating, while others cause a rapid and large spike in glucose. Eating a large bowl of pasta will raise your glucose more slowly than potatoes or corn, for instance, but the large quantity of carbohydrates may lead to a boost later because of the amount that must be stored. That's where the glycemic index and load come in, and we'll discuss those next.

Using the Glycemic Index

The *glycemic index* (GI) was developed to quantify how rapidly a carbohydrate is digested, which then dictates how much and how quickly insulin needs to be available to process it. The more rapidly a food is digested and absorbed, the faster it can end up as glucose in your blood. When you have a fully functional pancreas, the insulin released covers the increase in glucose from high-GI foods. When

130 • AGING WELL WITH DIABETES

you have diabetes of any type, however, it's harder to have the insulin waiting and ready to cover all the glucose with precision.

GI values go from 0 to 100. Glucose is a simple sugar with a GI of 100. Your GI for a particular food can vary since GI is affected by many different things. The macronutrient content of what you eat, how much fiber is in it, what starches exist, how it's prepared or cooked, its ripeness, and its acidity can all have an impact. Overcooking generally raises GI (so al dente pasta has a lower value), and highly acidic foods like vinegar slow down stomach emptying and absorption. Even letting your oatmeal get cold creates resistant starches that lower its GI.

Since it can vary so much, checking your glucose after eating is the best way to see the impact a meal or a food is uniquely having on you. The excessive intake of foods with a high GI value can lead to insulin resistance in most people, with and without diabetes. In overweight adults, insulin resistance has been shown to decrease when they eat a low-GI, whole-grain diet compared to a refined "white" one, and if you have type 2 diabetes, eating a diet with a GI of less than 40 has the potential to improve blood glucose, lower insulin resistance, reduce inflammation, drop cholesterol levels, and help you lose a few pounds to boot. If you don't have diabetes yet, a diet with a lower GI and fewer carbohydrates may actually prevent its onset.[14,15]

White potatoes naturally have a high GI, but the actual value depends on how you prepare them and what you eat them with (things that may slow down absorption). The GI of french fries is 75, but that's lower than the GI of the same potatoes not fried in oils that slow digestion. GI ranges vary among common foods (box 4.6).

Considering Glycemic Load

Particularly when you're eating carbohydrates, portion size matters. Related to the GI is something called *glycemic load* (GL), which takes

Box 4.6
GI Ranges and GI of Some Common Foods

High GI: 70–100

- Foods with white flour or added sugar, such as most breakfast cereals, pretzels, sugary candy, most crackers, and white bread

Medium GI: 56–69

- Sweet potatoes, rice (white, brown, basmati), oatmeal and other oat-based cereals, white sugar, sweet corn, bananas, raw pineapple, raisins, cherries, and multigrain or whole-grain wheat or rye bread.

Low GI: 0–55

- Most whole fruits, fructose (fruit sugar), legumes (beans), pasta (white or whole wheat), chickpeas and lentils, green vegetables, nuts and seeds, steak, hot dogs, poultry, fish, cream, cheese, sour cream, and many more

into account both the GI of a food and the total carbohydrates you get in a typical serving. Paying attention to your GL is even more important when you're trying to manage your blood glucose responses. There's no doubt that eating both high-GI and high-GL foods and meals can affect the efficacy of any insulin you have (natural or supplemental).

GL values go from 0 up. A high GL is 20 or more, while 11 to 19 is medium, and 10 or less is low. The GL gives you a measure of a food's carbohydrate density for each serving. You don't have to stick to just one serving: you can calculate the GL of any serving size for a single food, an entire meal, or an entire day's worth of food if you're counting your carbohydrates.

If the GL is over 20, you're getting a lot of carbohydrate in each serving, and if the spike in your glucose isn't immediate (because the

GI is lower), you'll still have to cover the total carbohydrate load over the next few hours (think huge plates of pasta: medium GI but very high GL). Limit your portion size when eating rice, pasta, beans, potatoes, or noodles to limit the overall GL of your meal. You can also choose slowly absorbed carbohydrates, not necessarily just a smaller amount of total carbohydrates.

Having a low GL usually means a food has a lower GI, but some exceptions exist. For instance, the GI of watermelon is 72, but per serving its GL is only 4 (but watch how many servings you eat since one serving is only about a cup). Popcorn has the same GI (72), but you can eat a lot to get to a single serving (four to five cups popped) with a GL of 8.

Legumes are rich in protein and fiber and have a lower GI. A low-GL, high-fiber diet also raises circulating levels of *adiponectin*, an anti-inflammatory hormone released by fat cells that can increase your insulin action and improve your blood glucose. A low-GI/GL diet plan results in weight loss as well.

Becoming More Sugar Conscious

In the GI section, you may have noticed that refined white sugar actually has a lower GI than a baked potato (because it's half fructose, half glucose), but the negative health effects of eating a lot of sugar and other refined carbohydrates can be significant since they lack essential nutrients (besides calories) and can be addictive as they release hormones like *dopamine* (in the brain's pleasure center). All ultraprocessed foods with a high fat, sugar (box 4.7), and fructose content and foods prepared at high temperatures can create *advanced glycation end products*, which accelerate liver injury and can lead to systemic inflammation. Refined sugar diets are often ill advised when people are trying to fight off cancer as well.

Box 4.7
Find the Hidden Sugars in Foods and Drinks

By law, manufacturers must list ingredients in order of descending weight, meaning that the first ingredient is the most prevalent in that product. If they hadn't come up with creative ways to list refined sugar, it would often be the first ingredient. In many products, companies add smaller amounts of four or five different sweeteners so they appear lower on the list of ingredients.

Look for the total "added sugar" on food labels, along with hidden-sugar equivalents. These include sucrose (table sugar), dextrose (glucose), high-fructose corn syrup, corn syrup, glucose, fructose, maltose, levulose, honey, brown sugar, and molasses.

You don't need to totally avoid fructose (fruit sugar) despite research suggesting that high-fructose corn syrup can cause a fatty liver. Simply avoid taking in too many empty calories made with any type of sugar or white flour. Be aware of which foods have them and don't go overboard on those. Your blood glucose will also likely benefit from cutting down on sugary drinks and fruit juices. Never drink more juice than you could consume in an equivalent amount of whole fruit—and eating six to eight whole oranges to equal a glass of juice would be a lot! Focus instead on foods higher in fiber, since those are usually lower in added sugars, fat, and calories.

Counting Your Calories, Not Just Carbohydrates

If you take insulin, you must guess how much you'll need to cover your meals and snacks—which can be a daunting task on a good day and nearly impossible on a bad one. Many individuals with diabetes, particularly mealtime insulin users, have learned to count the carbohydrates in their foods (usually their best guess) to match the total grams with the amount of insulin needed based on their unique carbohydrate-to-insulin ratio. Yours may be something like 30:1, meaning you need 1 unit of mealtime insulin for every 30 grams, but your ratio may vary with the time of day, types of carbohydrates, and recent or planned physical activity.

More recently, studies have proven what most of us insulin users have known all along, which is that even protein and fat in our foods can require some insulin to cover them. Some protein is converted into glucose (although more slowly than carbohydrates), usually three to four hours after you eat it.[16,17] The fat in your meals can also increase insulin needs (even when you eat the same amount of carbohydrates but just add in fat). Most fat is slow to be digested and may curb the rate at which other foods are converted into glucose as well, but it typically has no immediate impact on your blood glucose peak after meals. In other words, all calories can raise blood glucose, not just those from carbohydrates. You'll need to keep that in mind to dose insulin correctly if you take it.

Drinking to Keep the Doctor Away?

You've heard the saying, "An apple a day keeps the doctor away," but what about an alcoholic drink a day? It may as well! Research is being conducted all the time on the effects of drinking moderate amounts of alcohol, but the overwhelming majority of studies support the notion that drinking in moderation may lead to a longer life span than either drinking too much or not at all. It may be due to alcohol's impact on cardiovascular disease, which is still the leading cause of death among Americans. Moderate amounts of alcohol may increase levels of the "good" HDL cholesterol, increase blood flow to the heart, and improve insulin sensitivity while decreasing blood clots and artery spasms related to mental stress. Drinking does indeed help most individuals relax, and it may lower your risk of developing Alzheimer's disease.

So how much is a "moderate" intake of alcohol that could benefit your health? The lowest death rate from all causes occurs with one to two drinks per day (one for most women, two for most men). Death from all causes averages 16% to 28% lower among moderate drinkers than abstainers, but you can raise your mortality risk quickly by consuming more than the recommended amounts.[18] And consuming any alcohol is associated with a greater risk of breast cancer in women. The latest studies are suggesting that consuming even small amounts of alcohol regularly may raise your risk of other health issues as well, so the jury is still out on whether moderation or abstention may be better. Both of us know older individuals who have regularly consumed moderate amounts and lived to a ripe old age, though, so you have to consider both physical and mental health when deciding whether alcohol is appropriate as you age.

The health benefits of red wine—containing an antioxidant compound called *resveratrol* found in the skin of grapes—have been touted the most. The resveratrol, flavonoids, and anthocyanins found in winemaking grapes can fight cancer, heart disease, degenerative nerve diseases, and other ailments.[19] Grapes of all colors bestow health benefits, but red wine has more because many of these disease-fighting compounds are found in the grape skins.

When it comes to heart disease, it doesn't appear to matter which type of alcohol you choose to consume. To get as much resveratrol as you need from red wine, you'd likely have to consume more than the allowed number of drinks in any case. One older gentleman Dr. Colberg knew found that having two shots of whiskey at bedtime kept his morning blood glucose levels lower than when he missed drinking and wondered if he should keep up the habit. She said, "Of course!" (Whiskey's impact on the liver is to suppress glucose release.)

If you don't drink now, there is no need to start. In some cases, people need to completely avoid drinking alcohol, particularly if they have liver disease or memory problems. Taking certain medications may require abstinence from alcohol as well (such as many blood thinners). When in doubt, it's best to discuss this topic with your doctor and make sure the amount of alcohol you are consuming is okay for you personally.

It's a fine balance between taking in some alcohol and overimbibing, which can increase your risk of other health issues, including weight gain from the extra calories (seven calories per gram of alcohol). If you choose not to drink alcohol, simply focus instead on eating better, exercising more, and refraining from smoking to boost your health. In any case, taking in adequate (nonalcoholic) fluids on a daily basis is a surefire way to ensure you stay hydrated, prevent constipation, and maintain your urinary tract health.

PREVENT AND CORRECT NUTRITIONAL DEFICIENCIES

Your nutritional needs change with each passing decade, and the importance of getting adequate vitamins and minerals from your diet can't be overstated. One of the potential confounding factors in the onset of inflammation, insulin resistance, and type 2 diabetes is a lack of these *micronutrients*. Both dietary and bodily inadequacies are compounded by our decreased ability to absorb these nutrients from foods as we get older. Many vitamins and minerals are heavily involved in supporting the enzymatic pathways that make your metabolism work well—so deficiencies can result in a reduced ability to handle carbohydrates and keep your body healthy.

As you age, if you start eating small quantities and a less varied diet, you're at risk for deficiencies. If you eat fewer than 1,200 calo-

BOOST YOUR GUT HEALTH AND YOUR DIET • 137

ries per day, it's likely you're not meeting your micronutrient needs unless you're being very careful with your food selections. As a consequence, you need to know how to take in adequate nutrients for optimal health in your later years, especially when you have diabetes.

Getting More Vitamin D (and Calcium)

One of the most important vitamins is D, which is found in foods like fortified dairy products, nuts and seeds, and vegetable oils, but up to 90% is derived from sun exposure, making it the "sunshine vitamin." Vitamin D deficiencies are now widespread, a consequence of the excessive use of sunscreens to block ultraviolet (UV) rays in sunlight and less time spent outdoors, and they're also very common in people with all types of diabetes.

Vitamin D is the only vitamin that actually acts like a hormone and has the potential to affect every cell in the body through its pervasive receptors, and deficiencies have been linked to everything from the development of brittle bones to diabetes and certain types of cancer. It apparently may prevent some autoimmune diseases, diabetes, infectious diseases, heart disease, asthma, and neuropathy. Having enough vitamin D in your body also lowers your risk of dying from any cause.[20]

Although most active vitamin D is created in your body after exposure to sunlight, how much depends on the time of year since sunlight's UV strength varies with the season. You need to get sunshine on your face and hands for only a few minutes a couple of times a week to create what your body needs (depending on the time of year, of course, and where you live). Older adults don't create as much vitamin D in their skin with sunlight exposure, and receiving enough through diet alone is difficult.

Some foods naturally high in vitamin D include fish oils, fatty fish (like salmon), mushrooms, beef liver, cheese, and egg yolks, but sunshine likely increases levels more efficiently than eating these foods. You should probably take a vitamin D supplement if you don't get enough sun exposure and you're older.

Your bones have been thinning every year since you turned 25, and keeping your bone mass is now a top priority. That's where calcium comes in. At a minimum all women should consider eating more calcium-rich foods and possibly vitamin D supplements to prevent thin bones (*osteoporosis*) and fractures. After menopause you need around 1,300 mg of calcium daily. Calcium supplements used to be routinely recommended, but taking in excess calcium has been linked to an increased risk of heart disease. Experts now recommend that you get that amount daily by consuming calcium-rich foods.

Supplementation with at least 800 international units (IUs) of vitamin D is still prudent to ensure that your blood levels are high enough and that you absorb calcium efficiently (although supplements of up to 10,000 IU of vitamin D are now considered safe for most individuals with intact kidney function). Vitamin D levels are often low in people with diabetes. They can be measured in your blood, so consider asking your doctor to order that blood test for you.

In addition, cut back on your intake of phosphorus, a mineral abundant in colas containing phosphoric acid and many other foods and drinks. Balance your calcium intake with your phosphorus (one-to-one) to prevent calcium losses and bone thinning. Too much caffeine can have a similar effect on your bones, so avoid drinking colas or too much caffeinated coffee or tea. Also avoid excessive sodium intake.

Taking in Adequate B Vitamins

A whole family of water-soluble B vitamins are critically important to your metabolism since they are involved in the conversion of protein, fat, and carbohydrates into usable energy. Some of these are thiamine (vitamin B_1), riboflavin (B_2), niacin (B_3), pantothenic acid (B_5), pyridoxines (B_6), folate (B_9), and cobalamin (B_{12}). These are widely distributed in plant and animal foods, with the exception of vitamin B_{12}, which is only found in animal sources (vegans often need to take a B_{12} supplement to avoid pernicious anemia).

Deficiencies of some of the B vitamins are more common in people with diabetes, including thiamine, B_6, and B_{12}. Supplementing with thiamine (B_1), as well as with vitamin D, may improve insulin sensitivity.[21] Vitamin B_6 may prevent the formation of the advanced glycation end products associated with diabetes complications. Vitamin B_{12} deficiency is common with metformin use (see step 5), which can deplete this vitamin over time. Symptoms of nerve damage may be reversible with vitamin B_{12} supplements. A lack of it has also been associated with lower bone density in the spines of women and the hips of men.

Make sure your daily diet contains at least 100% of all the B vitamins, and consider taking at least a general B vitamin supplement. These are generally harmless because excess B vitamins are just peed out, but you also don't need to take megadoses. Taking in too much folate via supplements may actually mask a vitamin B_{12} deficiency and cause nausea. If you take metformin, invest in inexpensive multiple B vitamin supplements to combat potential deficiencies.

Otherwise, eating a balanced diet with adequate amounts of whole grains, vegetables (particularly the dark-green leafy ones), legumes, nuts, seeds, and healthy proteins will ensure you get plenty of the rest. Avoid eating too many highly refined foods or those containing table sugar, which usually have few of these vitamins left in them.

You may want to talk to your doctor about specifically supplementing with thiamine or *benfotiamine*, a lab-made version of this vitamin with additional antioxidant properties; both have been used to treat neuropathic pain. They may also prevent other diabetes complications, improve insulin action, and lower your cholesterol levels.

Getting Other Important Minerals

The American population as a whole is likely deficient in the mineral magnesium, which is involved in over 300 enzymatic pathways. It regulates energy production, the synthesis of DNA and RNA, protein formation, and bone health because it facilitates the enzymes and pathways that make these processes work. It affects blood pressure, regulates the rhythm of your heart, and prevents muscle cramps, and deficiencies have been associated with high blood pressure, stroke, plaque formation and heart disease, abnormal heart rhythms, altered blood fats, platelet stickiness, inflammation, oxidative stress, asthma, chronic fatigue, and depression. Low magnesium levels in adults with diabetes are also associated with eye disease and nerve damage.[22]

Look for magnesium in many foods but particularly in seafood; nuts; dark-green leafy vegetables like spinach, kale, and various species of lettuce; bananas; whole grains; legumes; and dark chocolate. If you're having frequent muscle cramps, you may be deficient in magnesium. You may lose magnesium through urinating more when your blood glucose is elevated, which may explain why deficiencies are more common in people with diabetes. Particularly if your blood glucose management could be better, you may want to consider taking a daily magnesium supplement of up to 350 mg, along with eating a more healthful diet. Taking too much magnesium can cause temporary diarrhea, but it's otherwise safe. If you have kidney failure, though, you may need to restrict your magnesium intake.

We need to mention a few other minerals that have a potential impact on diabetes. Chromium is known to have some positive effects on insulin efficacy. Selenium (found in abundance in Brazil nuts in particular) works with vitamin E to decrease oxidative damage. If you're deficient in zinc, your immune system may function suboptimally, and your insulin release may be impaired. Consider supplements if you are deficient in any of these minerals. In fact, most doctors agree that taking a multivitamin and mineral supplement daily may benefit elderly individuals, and they're usually relatively inexpensive and unlikely to harm you in any case.

Avoiding Excesses of Other Minerals

Sodium is the biggest concern for most people when it comes to the excess intake of minerals and/or electrolytes. Too much sodium in your diet can cause calcium loss from bones, not to mention its potential impact on your blood pressure if you're sensitive to it. To limit your sodium intake, cut back on visibly salted foods, canned products (unless they're salt-free or you wash your canned beans or corn with water), and highly processed prepackaged items.

A potassium deficiency may make you more sensitive to sodium, and people with the highest ratio of sodium to potassium in their diets have double the risk of dying of a heart attack and a 50% higher risk of death from any cause.[23] You may be able to avoid some of the downsides of excess sodium by simply making sure you have enough potassium in your diet (found in bananas, legumes, potatoes, broccoli, and many other fruits and vegetables).

Considering the Safety of Herbal and Natural Remedies

Aging brings its own set of physical and mental challenges, and up to 90% of people turn to complementary medicine and herbal remedies as they get older, including many potential herbal "cures." Everyone is looking for a way to manage or reverse what ails them, including common complaints like low back pain, arthritis and other joint pain, insomnia, depression, and aging itself. To be honest, most of them don't work, and both nutritional and herbal supplements are poorly regulated by the federal government. Some supplements contain none of what they say they do, and many remedies are based on unproven scientific theories or mechanisms. Just be careful if you go down this route as you never know what you're getting.

Some herbal medicines have been shown to be somewhat effective in the treatment of certain diseases, but few have become mainstream or widely accepted in medical circles. For instance, we do know that alpha-lipoic acid can help with painful diabetes-related neuropathy, but more clinical trials are needed to establish safe and effective dosing. Many have tried glucosamine for arthritic joints, with limited success. Ginger is sometimes used in the treatment of certain causes of vertigo.

When choosing herbal remedies or supplements, understand that having "herbal" or "natural" on the label doesn't mean a product is harmless. Some may actually harm you. It has been noted that certain forms of ginseng (used for dementia) can raise blood pressure, and mugwort can cause dermatitis (skin inflammation).

Let's take that last one as an example. Mugwort, a flowering plant native to northern Europe, Asia, and parts of North America, is used for anxiety, fatigue, constipation, diarrhea, depression, and epilepsy, just to name a few conditions. It can also cause allergic reactions, including a whole-body reaction called *anaphylaxis* that can lead to death if not treated immediately. Studies have shown that people allergic to celery (like Dr. Colberg), birch, or carrot should be cautious with mugwort because it's linked to "celery-mugwort-spice syndrome," a typically milder allergy that in rare cases can lead to anaphylaxis. (Dr. Colberg experienced a life-threatening anaphylactic response to celery root in the past, so she won't be trying mugwort anytime soon.)

Other "natural" supplements can interact with prescribed medications, potentially causing side effects or negating the benefits of the medication. People have died from taking herbal preparations containing heliotropium while also taking a prescribed barbiturate. No evidence exists to show how these supplements or herbs interact with current diabetes medications, so be extra careful with taking them. Always let your doctor know about any herbal or "natural" supplements you use, especially if you take any prescription medications.

Dr. Munshi typically tells her patients to avoid herbs in capsule form because we have no way of knowing their strength or what else is added to them. Because of that we don't know if they interact with any other meds they are taking. She tells them to eat herbs and spices like turmeric, garlic, ginger, and cinnamon in their natural forms.

Aging successfully and thriving are as much about your diet as they are the first three steps we covered (including getting enough physical activity). You know you need plenty of fiber to boost the good bacteria in your gut, and that will go a long way toward ensuring your lasting health. It also can't hurt to get more of the healthy omega-3 fats in your diet, take in plenty of protein, focus on eating more plants in general, and correct any deficiencies you may have. Even an alcoholic beverage (if you're female) or two (if you're male) daily may speed you on your way to better health. If nothing else, just following this step should help you feel more energetic, experience fewer illnesses, and continue aging more successfully.

CHAPTER FIVE

Step 5: Take a Medication Inventory

Are your many prescriptions weighing you down? When you're older and have diabetes, it is very likely that you're taking more than one prescribed medication. It's about time you look at what you're taking and whether you need all those meds. This step is all about avoiding "polypharmacy" (that is, taking multiple medications, or "meds" for short) to cut down on the potential for negative interactions between them. Some meds can lead to weight gain, cause insulin resistance, or change over time with regard to their impact on you.

Make a complete list of your current meds—including any over-the-counter ones and supplements—and take it to every medical visit to ask your health care team if you can safely reduce the dosage of some or eliminate others entirely. To ensure your optimal health, ask about new medications that may take the place of old (box 5.1).

MANAGE YOUR MEDICATIONS

We've been focusing on what a healthier lifestyle can do for you, but there is a time and a place for meds that may help manage your

Box 5.1
Step 5: Take a Medication Inventory

- What's old
  - Taking, and expecting to take, many different medications to treat all your ailments as you age
  - Never asking your doctor if any of your medications can be discontinued or if smaller doses may work
- What's new
  - Minimizing how many medications you take as you age to avoid drug interactions that require more treatments
  - Learning more about how prescription and over-the-counter medications and supplements may interact with one another
- What you should be doing
  - Talking with your health care team about ways to simplify your medication regimen, especially if you take four or more daily prescribed meds
  - Always having your current list of meds handy for your doctors and including any over-the-counter medications, herbs, and supplements

chronic ills. These can be naturally occurring or man-made and include prescription meds, caffeine, alcohol, nicotine, and over-the-counter pain relievers, along with illegal substances like cocaine or marijuana (which may be legal, depending on where you live) and herbal products such as saw palmetto and mugwort. Drugs are not just what the doctor prescribes for you. Many of these may cause unexpected or unpleasant side effects from drug interactions or allergies (box 5.2).

146 • AGING WELL WITH DIABETES

> **Box 5.2**
> **Insight from Dr. Munshi**
>
> As we get older and have more doctor visits, medications are often added but rarely taken away. As a geriatrician, when I see a new patient, I am more likely to remove some meds than to add more.
>
> Let me give you an example. One of my patients came in with high glucose levels, even after his metformin dose had been increased to maximum levels. He had also developed Parkinson's symptoms. During our visit, he had to run to the bathroom to throw up. I didn't see any obvious signs of Parkinson's, but he was on a lot of meds.
>
> When teasing out the timeline, I determined that his metformin had been increased rapidly (by another doctor), which can cause gastrointestinal side effects like nausea, vomiting, and a lack of appetite. For those symptoms he had been prescribed metoclopramide, which often has side effects that mimic Parkinson's disease. Because of those new symptoms, he had received even more meds, this time for Parkinson's (which he didn't actually have). This scenario, in which more meds are prescribed to counter the side effects of other meds, is very common—and one that everyone should try to avoid.

Using Medications Safely

You can take some precautions to make managing your medicines safer. If you're taking many meds at various times each day, you may want to use a weekly pill sorter that has separate sections for every day of the week. If you take your meds more than once a day, have separate sorters for different times of day. Here's more advice about what you should or shouldn't do when it comes to your meds.

DO all of the following:

- DO include your over-the-counter treatments, herbs and supplements, vitamins and minerals, and drug allergies on your list of prescribed meds.

- DO read the pill labels and follow the instructions exactly for pill timing and dosing listed on your prescription containers.
- DO ask for container labels with print large enough for you to read; if it's too small, you can either use a magnifying glass or take a picture with your phone and enlarge it.
- DO ask your pharmacy to send you medications in preorganized "bubble packs" if you are unable to read instructions properly.

DON'T do any of the following:

- DON'T put your meds into unmarked containers or those labeled for other meds.
- DON'T use meds that have expired; check with your doctor about getting a new prescription if they're past their "use by" date.
- DON'T share your meds with anyone else or take someone else's prescription meds (especially if you weren't prescribed that med by a health care provider).

Managing Polypharmacy (Five-Plus Prescriptions)

By definition, "polypharmacy" is when you take five or more meds daily. Technically, you're already experiencing *minor polypharmacy* when you take two to three meds daily and *moderate* when it's three to four.[1] Is taking a lot of prescribed medications a problem for Americans? According to a 2021 *Consumer Reports* survey, more than half of Americans take at least one prescription med daily, with the average person actually taking four.[2] Americans compose only 5% of the world's population yet take 50% of its prescription meds. Nearly 9 out of 10 older Americans have at least one prescription.

You'd think with all the meds that Americans would be the healthiest population on earth ... but that's far from true. More people than ever are being treated not only for diabetes but also for other chronic conditions like high cholesterol, high blood pressure (*hypertension*), and depression.

When you withdraw a medication that someone has taken for a long time, it makes them uncomfortable. But it can actually help in the long run when warranted. At the same time, if you do need to take many meds to address and manage your conditions, don't despair. Be thankful that we have so many options approved by the US Food and Drug Administration (FDA) now to help us remain healthy as we grow older. Meds aren't our enemies—just taking the wrong ones is!

So let's talk about how many is too many and how your meds may actually be causing you harm. As you age, it's common to have more than one health condition that needs treatment. Taking too many meds can lead to a vicious cycle of being prescribed more meds to counteract side effects from those you're already taking. Side effects from drug interactions can occur, even if you take as few as two meds a day. It's possible that some of your symptoms are the result of interactions of your multiple meds—like the scenario Dr. Munshi described.

If you take five or more medications, it's time to talk with your doctor about what you're currently on, including any supplements, such as herbals, over-the-counter medications, vitamins, minerals, and so on. Don't let your "cures" be part of the problem when it comes to treating your health conditions. If it's possible to cut back, you should. But only do so with the guidance of a doctor who is aware of your conditions and all the products you take to manage them.

Your Risk for Adverse Reactions and Side Effects

Certain factors increase your risk of having adverse reactions to and side effects from some of the meds you've been prescribed. In short, your age, genes, number of meds, doses, history of reactions, and hospitalization all contribute to your risk for adverse outcomes.

- **Age:** your risk of adverse events increases with advancing age.
- **Genes:** certain genetic traits make you more prone to drug interactions.
- **Daily meds:** the more you take, the greater the chance of side effects and/or adverse interactions between drugs.
- **Doses:** almost 80% of adverse drug reactions are related to dosage.
- **History:** if you have ever experienced an adverse reaction to any drug, your risk of reacting to another is higher.
- **Hospitals:** when you are given a drug while in the hospital, make sure it is *your* prescribed med since mistakes, unfortunately, are common in hospitals.

All drugs are metabolized in your liver and your kidneys. Their ability to process them quickly may decline as you age, meaning that drugs can hang around in your body for some time. In some cases, drugs accumulate in your fat tissue and are released later—when you're not expecting it—after you lose a few pounds. In short, a dose that may have been safe for you when you were 20 may be too much when you're only as old as 50 or 60. It's possible to have drug interactions even if you're only taking two meds.

Dr. Munshi also tells her patients that "the effects of drugs happen in everyone, but side effects occur only in a few." It's important to understand any possible side effects so you can recognize them if you do have them. But don't avoid taking a med because your friend or neighbor had some side effects. That may or may not happen to you as well. In most cases side effects are possible, not probable.

As a geriatrician, Dr. Munshi sees a lot of inappropriate care of older patients near the end of their lives, not because clinicians aren't trying to help or aren't paying attention but simply because they don't know what to do. We now understand how to manage individual conditions like heart disease, hypertension, high cholesterol, kidney disease, and more. When multiple conditions exist in the same person, however, it may not be appropriate to treat them as individual and unique conditions. Overall, a comprehensive and more holistic approach is needed, and that is what geriatricians (like Dr. Munshi) are trained to do (box 5.3).

Box 5.3
When Seeing a Geriatrician May Benefit You

For day-to-day problems and acute illnesses (like the flu or bronchitis), your family practitioner or internist is fine to see, and they can refer you to a specialist if needed. If you are over 65 years of age, you would probably benefit from seeing a *geriatrician*—that is, a doctor who specializes in the medical care and treatment of older adults. Since they specialize in health related to aging, geriatricians may be more knowledgeable than your usual doctor when advising you about medication use, providing the care you need, and helping you prevent future problems.

If you are over 70, you may want to seek out the care and medical advice of a geriatrician, if you are able to find one in your area, if the following applies to you:

- You take five or more medications daily
- You have multiple medical problems that may need a more holistic approach to treatment
- You are fatigued frequently or all the time
- You are having memory problems
- You are having falls for unexplained reasons
- You are feeling sad for no reason or for longer periods of time
- You struggle to complete daily self-care activities (e.g., showering, fixing meals)
- You are unhappy with the answers and advice from your regular physician

It's imperative that even nursing-home directors, nurses, clinical pharmacologists, and others who work directly with older populations know how to work with patients with diabetes and prediabetes since they are so prevalent in older adults. These clinicians and other professionals need to adopt strategies to help minimize the risk of hypoglycemia. This may include replacing a sliding-scale insulin-dosing regimen with more appropriate ones and doing a medication roundup.

Aging-related changes in drug effectiveness or new side effects may not happen overnight. Even if you've taken a certain med daily for decades, its effects may wane over time. When you start on a new med for the same health issue (such as a second blood pressure drug), the effectiveness of the first one or your response to it may also change. Some alterations in your responses over time occur not due to aging alone but due to having a diseased heart, liver, or kidneys. For meds you only use on occasion (e.g., antihistamines, sleeping pills, or pain relievers), be aware that your body may react differently to them with each passing year. Some drugs are better to avoid as you age (see appendix C), and potential drugs interactions should be monitored (appendix D).

Taking Medications as Prescribed

If your pill labels provide specific instructions about taking with meals or without food, follow them. Some must be taken with food to decrease the chance of stomach irritation, while others should be taken at least one hour before eating or two hours after meals to improve their absorption. In addition, always discuss dose changes with your doctor, and don't decide to alter them yourself. Even subtle changes in your doses can cause unwanted or dangerous side effects.

The cost of meds is also a factor for many older individuals. Discuss cost openly with your doctor because there may be cheaper alternatives, such as generic drugs, that can cut your costs whether you have insurance coverage or not. Your doctor's office usually doesn't know what drugs your insurance covers specifically, but if a generic medication will fit the bill, it can be indicated on your script. Ask about older drugs as well; just because a drug is newer doesn't mean it's more effective or better for you than an alternative cheaper, proven option.

Adding Medications on Your Own (Be Careful)

Nonprescription (over-the-counter) meds and some herbal supplements can still act as drugs or interact with other medications in negative ways. Always check with your doctor if you're planning to take anything else. Even nonprescription cold medicines or decongestants raise your chances of having an adverse reaction. For example, decongestants may worsen bladder problems from an enlarged prostate, antacids taken in excess can interfere with drug and vitamin absorption, and aspirin is well-known to prevent normal blood clotting.

Again, don't think that just because something is touted as "natural" or is an herbal preparation that it can't have any side effects or interactions. Saint John's Wort, an herbal remedy often used for mild depression, can interact with prescription medications for depression and make them less effective.[3] If you're taking medications intended for mental health purposes, be sure to mention those to your doctor, and check any counterindications when adding in a supplement.

WHAT YOU NEED TO KNOW ABOUT DIABETES MEDICATIONS

Picking the best medications to treat diabetes—type 2 in particular—has never been more complicated. When we both started working in the diabetes world, just one main class of drugs was available (sulfonylureas that increase insulin release from the pancreas), along with injected insulin, and no other options to lower blood glucose. Today there are multiple new classes of meds that target various bodily tissues, from your pancreas to your liver and kidneys. Sometimes knowing which to use can be difficult.

The good news is that many of the newer meds available to treat diabetes appear to have benefits over and above just lowering your blood glucose. For example, some from two of the newer classes of meds (incretin mimetics and SGLT-2 inhibitors—more on these in the next section) can lower your risk of heart attack, heart failure, and even hospitalization merely by being on them.[4,5]

It can help to learn more about the different categories of meds (since more drugs in certain classes of meds are being approved every day, which only confounds things further). In addition, various types of insulins can be given but may need adjusting based on lifestyle changes and the use of other medications.

Understanding Oral Diabetes Medications

Most pills to treat diabetes are intended for use by people with type 2 diabetes or prediabetes, not type 1 diabetes. Each class of meds targets different tissues in your body, including the pancreas (to increase insulin release), liver (to decrease blood glucose release), muscles (to make them more insulin sensitive), gut (to slow down the absorption of carbohydrates), and kidneys (to release excess glucose in the urine).

If you are newly starting any meds or increasing the dose, you may experience various side effects, such as stomach queasiness or diarrhea. In such cases try taking them with food, if recommended, to see if that helps. If your side effects remain bothersome, talk to your doctor about switching meds or lowering the dose.

The goal of all these oral meds is to manage blood glucose levels. If you make certain lifestyle changes—as we discussed in steps 3 and 4—it may be possible for you to lower your dosages or get off some of these meds entirely. Luckily, nowadays most of these oral meds don't increase the risk of hypoglycemia. Only those that stimulate the pancreas to release insulin (sulfonylureas and meglitinides) have any significant effect on your blood glucose responses, especially when you exercise. Some oral meds are used "off-label" by people with type 1 diabetes as well (such as metformin to lower insulin resistance and others that cause you to pee out extra sugar).[6] So let's take a look at the different classes of oral meds and how they work to lower blood glucose (table 5.1).

Alpha-glucosidase Inhibitors

This class of meds has two choices, Precose or Glycet, which work by slowing your digestion of carbohydrates after eating. They won't work if your digestion is slowed by a diabetes-related complication called *gastroparesis* (central nerve damage). Some newer classes of medications (like DPP-4 inhibitors and incretins) are more commonly prescribed since they slow digestion as well.

Biguanides (Metformin)

Metformin is the generic name of the only medication in this class. It's the most widely used drug for type 2 diabetes, prediabetes, and other insulin-resistant states. It's best for keeping your liver from overproducing glucose overnight, and it also improves insulin sensitivity in your muscles and your liver. If your morning glucose levels are high, then this med is one of your best choices. It's also possible to take it with other diabetes meds.

DPP-4 Inhibitors and Incretin Mimetics

Relevant to your gut health (step 4), the class of meds called DPP-4 inhibitors, or *gliptins*, work with gut hormones, natural enzymes, and your body's own insulin to lower blood glucose (DPP is short for

Table 5.1. Oral Diabetes Medications and How They Work

Medication class	Marketed as	How they work
Alpha-glucosidase inhibitors	Glyset, Precoset	Slow carbohydrate digestion in the gut; lower blood glucose spikes after meals
Biguanides	Metformin (generic), Glucophage (XR), Glumetza, Riomet	Decrease glucose release from the liver; increase liver and muscle insulin sensitivity
Combination therapies	Avandamet, Avandaryl, Duetact, Glucovance, Glyxambi, Janumet (XR), Jentadueto (XR), Juvisync, Kazano, Kombiglyze XR, Synjardy, etc.	Combine the effects of two or more medications in each pill
DPP-4 inhibitors (gliptins)	Januvia, Nesina, Onglyza, Tradjenta	Inhibit DPP-4, which normally breaks down the gut hormones called GLP-1 and GIP; improve insulin action; lower glucagon
Incretin mimetics* (also see the injectable versions)	Rybelsus (oral version of Ozempic)	Stimulate insulin release; inhibit the liver's release of glucose; delay emptying of stomach
Meglitinides	Prandin, Starlix	Stimulate beta cells to release insulin only to cover meals
SGLT-2 inhibitors	Brenzavvy, Farxiga, Invokana, Jardiance, Steglatro	Prevent kidneys from reabsorbing glucose; cause glucose loss through urine above ~180 mg/dL
Sulfonylureas	Amaryl, DiaBeta, Glucotrol, Glynase, Glycron (all second generation)	Promote insulin release from the pancreas; some may increase insulin action
Thiazolidenediones or glitazones	Actos, Avandia	Increase insulin sensitivity in muscles

"dipeptidyl peptidase"). Specifically, they block DPP-4 to increase the levels of two *incretin* (gut) hormones known as GLP-1 and GIP. These incretins regulate blood glucose homeostasis after you eat— and we'll discuss them more under the noninsulin injectable meds (although the GLP-1 agonist called Rybelsus is an oral version of these injectable incretins mimetics). DPP-4 inhibitors may also help preserve the ability of the pancreatic beta cells to make insulin.

Meglitinides

This class of *meglitinides* contains only two drugs, Prandin and Starlix, which work quickly to cause insulin release for a short duration. You take them before eating to prevent major postmeal spikes. If one of your main issues is your blood glucose rising sharply after you eat, you can benefit from these medications as long as your pancreas retains its insulin-making capacity. Watch out for glucose lows if you take a pill before a meal and exercise soon afterward, but only in the first hour or two when your insulin levels are higher.

SGLT-2 Inhibitors

This more recent class of meds (*sodium-glucose cotransporter-2 inhibitors*) causes a loss of excess blood glucose through the urine. Your kidneys filter a lot of glucose daily, but it gets resorbed back into your bloodstream. When you take these meds and your blood glucose rises above 180 mg/dL, excess glucose spills over into your urine and gets peed out. The extra sugar in your urine can increase your risk of yeast and urinary tract infections. When people with type 1 diabetes take these meds (off-label), they have an increased risk of *diabetic ketoacidosis* (elevated levels of ketones in the blood associated with insulin deficiency).[7] You may lose some weight with these meds since you're losing some glucose calories in your urine. They can lower your blood pressure and cause dehydration as well.

A potential positive side effect of these meds is better preservation of your kidney health and prevention of heart failure.[8]

Sulfonylureas

The original pills created to treat type 2 diabetes are in a class called *sulfonylureas*. They work by directly stimulating your pancreas to release more insulin—if it can—and are ineffective if your pancreas can't do that. The newer-generation sulfonylureas have fewer side effects and are less likely to cause hypoglycemia than the original ones in this class. Overall, sulfonylureas are less expensive than many meds in the newer classes, but they are completely reliant on your remaining insulin-making ability, which can decrease over time even in people with type 2 diabetes.

Although all medications from this class carry a high risk of hypoglycemia, some have a higher risk than others. Glucotrol (and generic versions of it) has no active metabolites and has the lowest risk of hypoglycemia with impaired kidney function. You may have to monitor for low blood glucose with these meds, particularly around physical activity and especially if you use the older-generation versions (e.g., Diabinese, Orinase), which stick around in your body longer.[9] The second-generation pills (Amaryl, DiaBeta, Glucotrol, Glynase, and Glycron) don't last as long and are preferred for use in older adults.

Thiazolidinediones

Called TZDs for short, thiazolidinediones work to make your muscles more sensitive to insulin ("insulin sensitizers"). They have some potential untoward side effects, though, like weight gain, bone fractures, and swelling of the feet and ankles, and you can't use them if you have heart failure, leg edema (swelling), or anemia. With all the adverse reactions, they are not prescribed as often as in the past.

Combination Pills

Even if you start out with only one oral medication (see table 5.1), it's common to end up taking others as well. Combination drugs that allow you to take just one pill are popular for that reason. Glucovance combines a sulfonylurea and a biguanide, and Avandamet is a combination of a glitazone (Avandia) and metformin. Some of the newer medications are available combined, such as DPP-4 and SGLT-2 inhibitors together in Glyxambi (Tradjenta and Jardiance) and Synjardy (metformin and Jardiance). New combinations seem to be coming out frequently, so expect many more weirdly named and hard-to-pronounce and -remember versions to come. Watch out for the cost when using combination drugs, though. On the one hand, you may only have to pay one copay instead of two; on the other hand, it may end up being more costly than taking two generic meds separately.

Understanding Noninsulin Injectable Diabetes Medications

Insulin is not the only injectable medication used to treat diabetes. Two other classes of meds are injected for type 1 and type 2 diabetes. One of them (amylin) replaces a hormone secreted with insulin, and the other class (incretin mimetics) affects gut hormones released when you eat (table 5.2).

Table 5.2. Injectable (Noninsulin) Medications and Actions

Class of medication	Marketed as	How they work
Amylin	Symlin	Works with insulin to limit glucose spikes for three hours after meals
Incretin mimetics	Adlyxin, Bydureon, Byetta, Mounjaro, Ozempic (oral: Rybelsus), Trulicity, Victoza	Stimulate insulin release by acting like the incretins GLP-1 and GIP; inhibit the liver's release of glucose; delay emptying of the stomach

Amylin

Amylin is a hormone usually cosecreted with insulin, so if your pancreas no longer makes insulin, you are missing this hormone. An injectable replacement was approved as Symlin, which can be used by anyone on insulin (type 1 and type 2 diabetes). Symlin, together with insulin, slows down the rate at which your blood glucose rises after meals. As an added bonus, it can cause weight loss since you may feel full sooner during a meal when taking it. Its biggest drawback is its ability to cause gastrointestinal problems like nausea and vomiting and even severe lows.[10] Dr. Colberg has known some active individuals with type 1 diabetes over the years who experienced what they called "Symlin lows," when their blood glucose would not rise no matter how much they ate. If you have a diabetes-related complication called *gastroparesis* affecting your digestion, you shouldn't use Symlin.

Incretin Mimetics

GLP-1 and GIP are naturally occurring *incretins,* or substances produced in the intestines when you eat. They normally work by promoting the release of insulin from your pancreatic beta cells and blocking the release of glucose-raising glucagon from your alpha cells. Medications in this class mimic the actions of incretins primarily by inhibiting DPP-4, an enzyme that breaks down incretin hormones before they have time to work effectively (DPP-4 inhibitors are a class of oral medications).

These mimetics are injected daily or once weekly—depending on which one you use—and one version can be taken as a pill (Rybelsus). Since they delay digestion and make you feel full sooner, they are one of the hottest medications on the market to help anyone lose weight (marketed to the general public for obesity as Wegovy and Zepbound). Their main downside is the potential for gastrointestinal symptoms like nausea.

Understanding Insulin Use

People with type 1 diabetes have lost all or almost all of their ability to make insulin and have to replace it using injections, an insulin pump, or an inhaler (one inhaled version is available). Some with type 2 diabetes also take insulin because they cannot produce as much as they require. In either case some lifestyle changes may lower the amount of insulin needed, and that's always a good thing. Many centenarians (people aged 100 years and older) have naturally low insulin levels with normal blood glucose levels, meaning they are very insulin sensitive. High levels of circulating insulin are associated with a whole host of chronic health problems and are best avoided. Even thin older people can have high levels of insulin resistance, though, due to low muscle mass and a relatively larger fat mass.

If you have type 2 diabetes and take insulin, you may be able to decrease your doses with improvements in your food choices, physical activity, body weight, and more. Individuals with type 1 diabetes can also lower their insulin needs through diet and exercise, although they'll always need to replace some missing insulin. If you develop type 1 as an adult (about half of those diagnosed with diabetes as adults, even though it used to be considered a juvenile disease), your insulin needs often stay low for much longer than if you were diagnosed in your younger years.

Depending on the type of insulin you take, it starts lowering your glucose at different times (onset) before reaching a maximal (peak) value and lasts based on its formulation (duration). Most current insulins have been modified slightly (creating insulin analogues) and bound with other substances to vary their onset and duration. Let's talk more about the types of insulin and how they are used (table 5.3).

Table 5.3. Insulins and Their Onset, Peak, and Duration Times

Insulin	Onset	Peak	Duration
Afrezza	12–15 minutes	35–45 minutes	2.5–3 hours
Admelog, Apidra, Humalog, NovoLog, Lyumjev	5–30 minutes, varies by insulin	0.5–1.5 hours	3–5 hours
Regular (R)	30–60 minutes	2–5 hours	5–8 hours
N (NPH)	1–2 hours	2–12 hours	14–24 hours
Basaglar, Lantus, Rezvoglar, Semglee, Toujeo	1.5 hours	None	20–24 hours
Tresiba	30–90 minutes	None	Over 24 hours

Basal Insulins

About a third of your daily insulin requirements qualify as *basal,* or background, needs even if you do nothing but rest or sleep all day without eating. Your body uses this insulin for basic maintenance and bodily functions. It also allows your resting muscles to take up and store glucose as glycogen, your liver to regulate glucose uptake or release, and your fat cells to store excess calories.

To cover basal insulin needs, some insulins are formulated to be released slowly over hours to days. Nowadays, almost everyone with type 1 diabetes follows a basal-bolus insulin regimen, meaning they take basal insulin and cover meals separately with a different type or varied delivery of insulin. If you have type 2 diabetes, you may take only basal insulin or add shorter-acting types for food intake, as most with type 1 diabetes do. A newer once-weekly insulin, icodec (brand name Awigli), has been tested in people with type 2 diabetes and may be a viable alternative for some once if approved by the FDA (rejected in 2024, pending in 2025).[11]

Insulin pump users receive small doses of insulin to cover their basal needs all day long, based on how the pump is programmed. They use shorter-duration insulins rather than basal ones because delivery is continuous (usually every five minutes). Some people use both an injected basal insulin and insulin pumps to deliver basal insulin during extended exercise or other conditions.[12]

Basal insulins are injected usually only once daily, but it can depend on their duration and your individual needs and preferences. Although traditionally a once-daily basal insulin dose is given in the evening, as one ages it works better when injected in the morning. If you frequently experience low glucose levels in the morning, ask your doctor if taking your basal insulin at that time will work better for you. In general, the larger the dose, the longer it takes to be fully absorbed and available in your bloodstream. For this reason, some insulin-sensitive individuals who take very small basal insulin doses that technically should last 24 hours (like insulin-glargine, U-100) must take them twice daily (although not necessarily as two equal doses).

Bolus (Mealtime) Insulins

Insulin given to cover a meal or snack or for correction is considered *bolus*, or mealtime, insulin because it acts quickly and has a limited duration. As mentioned, these insulins are also used in pumps as basal insulin when delivered frequently during the day in small increments.[13] Among the insulins available, the differences in their onset and peak times are minimal, but all work more rapidly than regular human (Humulin R) insulin. People tend to prefer the action of one over another, but any can potentially cover eating and corrections.

The trick with bolus insulin is to estimate the correct dose and its timing to best cover the glycemic profile of the foods you're eating. As mentioned in the last step, more insulin may be needed to cover high-carbohydrate foods than lower-carbohydrate options, but the rate at which a food is digested and converted to glucose must also be considered when deciding on a bolus dose. It takes a great deal of trial and error to get it right, and it never happens all the time since the varied factors that affect your immediate insulin needs can change on a daily, and sometimes hourly or minute-by-minute, basis.

Insulin-Delivery Methods

How you choose to take your insulin is an individual decision, and there are multiple options nowadays. Some may work better for you than others, but in case you're unaware of their benefits and drawbacks, the following information might influence your decision:

- Insulin syringe and insulin pen needles come in different lengths; choosing a shorter one if you have less body fat can make insulin delivery more comfortable.
- Dosing using insulin syringes can be difficult if you have sight limitations or a lack of dexterity in your hands.
- Dialing an exact dose on a pen is easier than filling a syringe from an insulin vial to the correct amount (which can be difficult if you can't see well).
- Using insulin pens reduces the likelihood of giving yourself a dose of the wrong insulin when you use two types because each has its own unique injection pen.
- Many insulin "smart pens" have the ability to record the last dose and time given, eliminating the need to manually track and log insulin doses and glucose values.
- Smart pens include reusable insulin pens or smart cap/attachments that attach to a disposable, prefilled insulin pen.
- Insulin pumps use a small catheter placed under your skin to deliver basal and bolus insulin doses, but they typically have to be changed out every three days.
- One insulin pump is tubeless (Omnipod), but all the rest have tubes attached that you must keep from catching on things and away from sunlight.

164 • AGING WELL WITH DIABETES

- Insulin pumps must be programmed to give the correct basal and bolus doses, so you need to be smarter than your pump.
- Most pumps now include features such as "bolus insulin on board" calculations and bolus dose calculators, as well as varying patterns of bolus insulin delivery.
- Some pumps integrated with continuous glucose monitoring systems (see step 1) can now calculate basal doses for you based on your glucose values, but meal doses are left to the user.
- Like a functioning pancreas, insulin pumps provide insulin in small doses all day long, with bigger doses following eating.
- Temporary basal dosing can be programmed into pumps at any time, whereas altering basal insulin delivery with injected insulin is much harder.
- If you hate shots, with a pump you only have to endure one needlestick, when the infusion set is inserted, every three days.
- An insulin patch "pump" (V-Go) is now available and works well for people with higher insulin needs; changed daily, it gives insulin at a preset basal rate of 20, 30, or 40 units every 24 hours.
- The V-Go provides on-demand bolus dosing of up to 36 units every 24 hours in 2-unit increments, so it won't work well if you need smaller bolus doses.
- The only inhaled insulin option, Afrezza, comes with cartridges that administer only 4, 8, or 12 units at a time, which can be a problem if you need a smaller dose.
- Inhaling the dry powder that Afrezza uses can cause coughing or throat irritation in some people, and you can't use it if you have asthma or emphysema.

Insulin and Exercise Interactions

Because insulin is the only hormone released by the body (normally) that has a glucose-lowering effect (as opposed to the five that can raise it), too much insulin in your body during and after physical activities can easily result in low blood glucose. We already mentioned the oral meds that are more likely to cause exercise-related lows (sulfonylureas and meglitinides), but almost any type of insulin can.

Insulin levels in your bloodstream normally decrease when you're active (assuming you can make your own). When you take insulin, though, its delivery method and duration in your bloodstream can pose difficulties with keeping your glucose levels from dropping too low. Remember that muscle contractions themselves cause glucose uptake into active muscles and that insulin independently does the same—and the effect is additive.

We briefly discussed why this happens back in step 3, but let's talk more about how you can keep your blood glucose in balance when you're physically active. Exercising with low levels of insulin in your bloodstream will bring you a much more normal physiological response, and that is what you should aim for. Knowing when, how, and why to adjust your insulin doses can be critically important to managing your blood glucose.

Managing Insulin for Exercise

Much debate has centered around the optimal time to exercise with either type of diabetes. Since most with type 2 diabetes are not taking meds that increase their risk of exercise-related lows, being active following meals can help lower any spikes in blood glucose. For people taking mealtime insulin, insulin levels are highest and the hypoglycemia risk greatest immediately after meals.[14] Dr. Colberg always advises people that the best time to be active is when you can fit it into your daily life (otherwise, you may skip it).

That said, here are some things you should know about lowering the negative impact of insulin on blood glucose when you're active:

- The peak, onset, and duration of any insulins you take can have a big effect on your blood glucose responses (see table 5.3).
- Having only basal insulin "on board" while exercising will lead to a more normal response than insulin levels that are too high or too low.
- Exercising when your insulin levels are peaking—usually in the 2–3 hours after taking mealtime insulin—increases your risk of going low.[15]
- If you take only basal insulin or more than 2–3 hours have passed since your last bolus dose for a meal, snack, or correction, your risk of going too low decreases.
- If you use an insulin pump, you can prevent most lows by reducing your basal insulin delivery rates during exercise or disconnecting your pump for up to an hour at a time when active.
- If you exercise longer than an hour and remove your pump, you may have to briefly reconnect it and receive a small insulin dose every hour to prevent your glucose from going too high. Alternatively, you can use an injected basal insulin for coverage.
- It's also possible to decrease the basal insulin rate on your pump an hour or two before you start and keep it that way afterward for a time, depending on how long you're active and the intensity of the activity.
- Following physical activity, you may need less insulin for 2–72 hours afterward, depending on what you do and how long you stay active.
- If you inject your basal insulin, dosing twice a day gives you more chances to adjust your dosing to prevent exercise-related lows.
- You may need to lower both your bolus and your basal insulin doses after exercising in the short run and the longer term (if your training is consistent).

- Your insulin may act more quickly depending on where you inject it when you exercise; hot-tub use and vigorous massage around injection sites can have a similar effect.

Adjusting your insulin doses optimally before and after activities requires you to understand how insulins work and have some practice doing it. Start by cutting back by just a unit or two of insulin and make adjustments as you measure your body's response. Don't worry that it takes some trial and error to get closer to your target numbers. You may need to take lower insulin doses overall to compensate for being active regularly. If you're more active at certain times of the year, you may have to lower your insulin doses during those times and raise them at others. And keep in mind that when you're doing intense, near-maximal exercise—especially first thing in the morning before breakfast or any insulin—you may need to increase your bolus insulin rather than lower it.

If you're uncertain about how to adjust insulin doses or feel uncomfortable trying to handle it on your own, consult with your health care provider or seek out other resources (box 5.4). Doing so is particularly important if you begin to experience frequent lows related to your activities (see step 1 about preventing hypoglycemia) and are relatively new to being active. You can learn a lot from how others manage their glucose when doing various activities.

Box 5.4
More Physical Activity Guidance for Insulin Users

For additional guidance on how others change their insulin and/or food intake for a variety of activities, consult specific activity recommendations in Dr. Colberg's book *The Athlete's Guide to Diabetes: Expert Advice for 165 Sports and Activities* (Human Kinetics 2020). It also goes into much more depth about the physiology behind exercise and specific insulin adjustments.

168 • AGING WELL WITH DIABETES

If you eat extra before exercising, you may not need to adjust your insulin, or the needed changes may be less. For longer activities most people who use insulin have to lower their doses *and* eat more carbohydrate to compensate. If you know you're going to be active shortly after eating, consider reducing the carbohydrates you eat at that meal so you can cut back on your insulin without your blood glucose rising too high before you start. Try to keep your pre-exercise doses as small as possible (so they're absorbed faster and out of your body sooner).

UNDERSTANDING INTERACTIONS OF EXERCISE WITH OTHER MEDICATIONS

Insulin isn't the only prescription drug that can affect your ability to be more active when you have diabetes and are getting older (and possibly taking a lot of other meds). At this point, you may be taking meds for high cholesterol, high blood pressure, pain management, and other health issues. Let's talk about which have the greatest interactions, or no interaction at all, with your ability to be physically active. Also, always keep in mind that even if such interactions happen to someone you know, your body may or may not have the same response. Don't avoid taking certain meds that may help you just because others have had untoward interactions.

Statins and Muscle/Joint Health

Many people take *statins* to lower their overall and bad (LDL) cholesterol levels and reduce their risk of having a heart attack or stroke. A number of statins are currently available for use, the most common being atorvastatin (Lipitor) and rosuvastatin (Crestor); others include Simvastatin (Zocor), Pravastatin (Pravachol), and Lovastatin

(Mevacor). Like diabetes meds, some statins are combined with other meds for heart health, such as Caduet and Vytorin.

People with diabetes of any type have a much higher risk of having a cardiovascular event, and most medical professionals prescribe low- to moderate-dose statins for adults aged 40–75 with diabetes and an LDL cholesterol level between 70 and 189 mg/dL. You're even more likely to be prescribed one if you have known blood vessel disease, high blood pressure, or smoking as a risk factor. Nowadays, statins have been shown to have benefits, even in older age groups, beyond lowering total and bad cholesterol levels.

Although the benefits of statin use are seen in people of all ages with diabetes, they are not without potential drawbacks in some individuals. They can cause damage to muscles, muscle pain, and weakness during physical activity. Muscular conditions such as myalgia, mild or severe myositis, and rhabdomyolysis, although relatively rare, are much higher in people with diabetes.[16] Some people experience more exercise-induced muscle injury when on statins, particularly active older individuals. Dr. Munshi would advise that if you take a statin and experience symptoms such as muscle cramps or fatigue after exercising, talk with your doctor about potentially switching to another cholesterol-lowering drug.

Long-term statin use in rare instances may also affect the strength of the connectors (tendons and ligaments) around joints and predispose you to ruptures. Statin users have also been reported to have more spontaneous ruptures of both their biceps and Achilles tendons.[17] On the good news front, statins and metformin are being tested in large research trails to see if they can counter other age-associated declines in health, and metformin may act as a possible protectant against statin-related muscle symptoms.

Beta-Blockers

Beta-blockers are a class of prescribed meds used to treat high blood pressure and heart disease. Examples include Bystolic, Corgard, InnoPran XL, Levatol, Lopressor, Sectral, Tenormin, Toprol XI, Zebeta, and some generic brands. When it comes to exercise, any of these can potentially lower both your resting and exercise heart rates, making it harder to monitor your exercise intensity unless you do it subjectively (see step 3). From a diabetes standpoint, these meds can blunt your hormonal response to going low and increase your risk for more severe low blood glucose events. If you take beta-blockers, you should be aware of these effects; however, keep in mind all the benefits of beta-blockers for your health condition.

Diuretics

Known as water or fluid pills, *diuretics* cause you to urinate out extra bodily fluids and salt, which serves to lower blood pressure, relieve fluid from around your heart, and reduce ankle swelling. They fall into a few categories, including thiazides, loop diuretics, and potassium-sparing meds. While none are likely to have an impact on your diabetes management, they can lead to dehydration, especially if your blood glucose has been running above normal. Watch out for low blood pressure, dehydration, and dizziness during exercise if you use these meds.

Vasodilators

Taking a *vasodilator* like nitroglycerin improves the amount of blood flowing to your heart muscle during rest and exercise, which can relieve chest pain (*angina*). Just be aware that they can also cause your blood pressure to drop during exercise, which can make you feel dizzy or faint.

Blood Thinners

If you take aspirin or another blood thinner such as Coumadin, you should understand that they can make you bruise more easily or extensively if you suffer an exercise-related or athletic injury. You can exercise normally, though, and have nothing to worry about related to your blood glucose levels.

ACE Inhibitors and Others

ACE inhibitors (e.g., Capoten, Lotensin, Monopril, Vasotec, Zestril, and others) or angiotensin II receptor blockers (like Cozaar, Benicar, and Avapro) taken to lower blood pressure or protect your kidneys have no impact on exercise, although certain ACE inhibitors may lower your risk of an exercise-related heart attack. Meds like calcium-channel blockers, antidepressives, and pain blockers also do not affect it.

Corticosteroids

The only other med with the ability to affect your blood glucose is any type of corticosteroid—like prednisone or injections into inflamed joints—as these cause severe insulin resistance and the potential for blood glucose elevations.[18] Some people must take these medications frequently for breathing difficulties or inflammatory arthritis. If you get an athletic or overuse injury, have spinal stenosis, or experience another health condition that has to be treated with this class of meds, do what you can to keep your blood glucose levels as normal as possible.

Now that you know so much more about how to manage your medication regimens as you age with diabetes, it's time to move on to our next topic, your body weight. Many of the items discussed in these last three steps also influence body weight, so you may want to refer back to these after you read through the next step.

CHAPTER SIX

Step 6: Achieve Your Desired Body Weight

How many times over the years has your doctor told you to lose a little weight? In the middle years of your life, modest weight loss can prevent the onset of type 2 diabetes and other health problems, but during your later years, you may need to lose it carefully (if at all). Since having diabetes makes you more likely to drop the good kind of weight (that is, muscle instead of fat), you'll want to work to combat muscle loss if you plan on slimming down (refer back to step 3 on resistance exercise). Some fat-soluble medications can build up in your fat tissue, increasing your blood levels if you lose a lot of weight quickly, so you'll probably need to lower your overall doses to correspond with your new weight. It's also possible to have a depressed appetite as you age, and if you start losing muscle mass because of it, you'll need to work on eating more of the right foods to combat that (box 6.1). The good news is that making changes to your lifestyle can help you prevent or reverse some of these problems when you're older.

Although it is possible to lose weight at any age, several factors make it harder to lose the right kind of weight with age. Physical activity, one of the most important aspects of a healthy lifestyle, helps promote muscle maintenance, along with the loss of body fat.[1] Older

ACHIEVE YOUR DESIRED BODY WEIGHT • 173

Box 6.1
Step 6: Achieve Your Desired Body Weight

- What's old
  - Gaining weight as you get older and losing your muscle mass
- What's new
  - Fighting to keep or increase the amount of muscle you have (and possibly losing a few pounds—of fat only)
- What you should be doing
  - Talking with your health care team about ways to gain muscle mass and safely lose fat from the right areas and maintaining your new weight

---

people tend to have more aches and pains and to be more sedentary, which can result in either a loss of muscle mass or weight gain or both. But even if you are a regular exerciser and always have been throughout your life, you're losing some muscle over time. Starting in about your 30s, bodily changes related to the aging process cause us to start losing muscle (box 6.2). Since your muscles require more daily calories to maintain than your fat cells (which require very little), your metabolism and calorie needs can decline over time, making it easier to gain fat weight while you're losing muscle.

Blood levels of the sex hormones estrogen and testosterone decline when you hit menopause (women) or "andropause" (men) and can compound muscle losses and fat gains. Most women typically start entering menopause around their early 50s (the national average for age at menopause is 51 in the United States).[2] Once you've gone a full year without a menstrual cycle, you've reached it. For men, the levels of testosterone drop off noticeably, but this tends to happen somewhat later compared to when women lose estrogen.

Box 6.2
Insight from Dr. Munshi

Later in life, your body will have a smaller muscle mass and more fat even if the circumference of your arms and legs has remained the same over time. So your goal should be to keep or increase your muscle and possibly lose some fat. If you try to lose weight through dieting alone, however, you'll lose some muscle along with the fat. Exercise helps maintain muscle, which is as important as maintaining a healthy weight. But cardio exercise should be supplemented with strength training using weights, resistance bands and tubes, or body-weight exercises. Eating more protein—but not more calories—may also help build or sustain your muscles. The last thing you want to do for your health and mobility is end up underweight with less muscle mass.

FINDING YOUR IDEAL BODY WEIGHT

Just like Goldilocks, it can be challenging to find the right body weight as you age. What's too fat, or too thin, or just right? Is it the same for you now that you're older compared to your younger self? The goal isn't just the number on the scale but the way you maintain a healthy weight and the strength to go with it. The medical term for muscle wasting is *sarcopenia,* and you want to avoid that as much as possible, although some muscle loss with aging is inevitable. You're looking to achieve good muscle fitness, no matter your body weight, to help ensure that you spend your later years in better health and are able to do more of what you like.

Body Weight and Current Trends

While the United States became the fattest nation in the world during the 20th century, our average life span still increased by 27 years (we've backtracked a little due to COVID-19, however). In general, this statistic tells you that things are not always as they appear or as simple as we would like. Being slightly overweight—with *slightly* being the operative word—or gaining weight later in life as opposed to earlier in adulthood may actually improve your health and prolong your life.[3,4] Especially when you're over 60 years old, major weight loss is not recommended unless your weight puts you in the category of obese.

And in recent years, it's not just about body weight when over half of Americans report being on a diet of some sort. More than ever, we've been eating a particular diet or following a certain pattern, like "eating clean" or "mindful eating," to not only lose weight and look better but also to feel better. Some of these fads stem from the fact that nutrition information is so confusing and often conflicting: eat this, don't eat that, fat is good, fat is bad, eat protein, avoid carbohydrates, eat fewer calories, eat all the calories you want as long as they're not from carbs, and more.

The latest trend is using what were developed as blood glucose management medications as drugs for weight loss in the general population. In particular, the incretin mimetics discussed in step 5 are being marketed for weight loss: Wegovy (semaglutide), Saxenda (liraglutide), and Zepbound (tirzepatide). These meds are used in varying doses to treat type 2 diabetes with the trade names of Ozempic, Victoza, and Mounjaro, respectively. Zepbound is the newest med just approved for weight loss, and it combines GLP-1 and GIP (refer back to step 5 for a definition). As an added side benefit, they appear to be heart protective and improve blood pressure and cholesterol levels.[5,6]

Excitement about these particular meds has been high because they can help you lose as much as 20% of your total body weight, which exceeds what any prior weight loss drug on the market could offer. The demand for these meds by adults without diabetes has been unreal. As soon as the US Food and Drug Administration (FDA) approved Ozempic, the high demand for it as an off-label weight-loss drug grew so that for months it was hard to find for people with diabetes, and physicians had to prescribe alternate meds, at least temporarily.[7] Remember, though, that these meds are not without side effects, and weight regain (of two-thirds of the loss or more) often follows when people stop using them.[8]

When Weight Gain May Be Good

Body fat has become maligned, but its bad rap is not entirely deserved. Recent research has shown us how body fat is an active metabolic tissue. It produces some hormones—such as *adiponectin* and *leptin*—that help drive hunger and regulate food intake and metabolic rate. These can be altered by physical activity and other lifestyle changes.[9] Fat tissue also releases compounds called *cytokines*, which can contribute to systemic inflammation (refer back to step 2 for more about the causes and markers of inflammation).

We have traditionally blamed body-fat gains for the onset of insulin resistance and type 2 diabetes, but research clearly shows that you can normalize your blood glucose levels with a minimal weight loss of 5%–7% of your body weight. This is only about a 10-pound loss if you weigh 200 pounds and about a 15-pound loss if you weigh 300.[10]

Losing a pound of muscle weight, which is largely water, is often quicker and easier than dropping an equivalent amount of fat, so don't get discouraged. Slow weight loss usually results in a greater fat loss than rapid weight-loss techniques. Also, if you lack fat right below your skin's surface (subcutaneous fat—the "pinch an inch" type), you can develop *lipoatrophic diabetes* caused by having too little fat (and places to store excess calories effectively). So the presence of extra fat cannot be wholly responsible for prediabetes and type 2 diabetes.

Body fat also helps protect your internal organs, and fat around your hips helps cushion them from fractures if you take a fall. Fat also has an insulating effect and keeps you warm when it's cold outside. Our ability to thermoregulate—that is, keep our body temperature normal under environmental extremes—actually diminishes as we get older. If you feel cold all the time—in part because your metabolism has slowed and you're making less body heat—having more fat can help you feel warmer. It has also been noted that people with a higher amount of body fat—stored for later use under less abundant food conditions—survive long stays in the hospital and prolonged illnesses better than those who are closer to a normal weight or underweight.[11]

Overall, body fat may be associated with many health conditions, but it's not necessarily the direct cause of all that ails you (box 6.3). For example, when you start doing exercise training on a regular basis, your muscle cells not only become more insulin sensitive but you're also likely to lose some of your deep abdominal fat and lower your systemic inflammation, both of which have great health benefits.[12]

When Weight Loss Can Be Bad

When you're older, losing weight—unless it's intentional—has been shown to be associated with almost double the odds of dying, even if you are overweight or obese to start with and especially when you have diabetes. The risk of dying when you lose weight is also higher when you have heart disease.

Serious Health Problems

In older women, purposely losing weight may not always increase their risk of dying, but it more than doubles their risk of fracturing a hip, becoming frail, and having to enter a nursing home for care.[13,14] In some people, losing weight unintentionally or unexpectedly is the

Box 6.3
The Pros and Cons of Body Fat

Pros

- More cushion around the hips to prevent fractures from falls
- Insulating effect to keep you warmer
- Increased chance of survival during prolonged illnesses and hospital stays
- Not directly responsible for onset of type 2 diabetes
- May help maintain muscle in lower limbs due to carrying extra weight
- Limited amounts not shown to increase the risk of death from any cause
- Prevents lipoatrophic diabetes (from too little subcutaneous fat)

Cons

- Excess stress on lower extremity joints from extra weight
- Increased inflammation and insulin resistance risk with visceral (central) adiposity
- Greater risk of sleep apnea
- Bodily dissatisfaction
- Mobility issues and greater risk of muscle wasting if inactive
- Greater risk of nonalcoholic fatty liver disease
- Greater risk of dying associated with too much fat weight

sign of another serious health issue, such as cancer. If you're over 60 and lose weight without knowing why, check with your doctor to rule out any potential diseases that may be causing it. Generally, major weight loss is not advised once you reach the age of 60. If you're younger than 60, there's still time to work on preventing excess body weight—especially around your belly area, which can harm your health—by adopting a healthier lifestyle.

Loss Followed by Weight Regain

Another reason to avoid excess weight loss when you're older is that you invariably lose some muscle when you lose pounds, even with regular exercise. Weight cycling, or losing and then regaining weight, can leave you weaker and more prone to dying than never having lost the weight at all.[15] Basically, you probably lost some muscle and mostly gained back fat. If you are losing any body weight—whether you're trying to or not—it's essential to exercise to maintain your muscle mass.[16] In fact, physical activity is likely more important than how many calories you eat when it comes to maintaining a good body weight and your health.

Weight loss usually consists of about 75% fat and 25% muscle for the typical dieter, and regaining the weight—which is very common—results in 85% fat and 15% muscle gain. So you can end up 10% fatter and at the same weight (or higher) than before you lost any weight. If you go through these weight cycles (up and down) frequently, you may end up with too little muscle to move your body mass around, setting you up for a whole host of potential health problems just related to being less active. You could become a member of the "overweight and frail" disabled club.

There also appears to be a lasting impact on your resting metabolism from weight cycling over your lifetime. If you lose significant amounts of weight when younger and gain it back, your metabolism slows once you've regained it and likely remains slower. This was found in individuals who lost weight on TV shows such as *The Biggest Loser*. Once they regained weight, their metabolisms were slower than they were at their original weight, and the effects were maintained for years afterward.[17] Losing fat cells apparently tricks your brain into thinking you're starving, and for survival reasons your body slows its basal needs to hold onto those calories. If you were ever heavy (even if you're not as heavy now), you'll need to eat less to maintain the same weight.

Released Medications

You may not realize it, but some of your prescription meds are stored in your body fat, and significant weight loss may release those meds into your bloodstream. You may need lower doses of any meds you've been taking as a result, but chances are that simply losing weight will affect your dosage needs more than any potential release of fat-soluble drugs from fat loss. Be sure to discuss your medications with your doctor as you lose weight or if you plan to diet.

Protein Energy Malnutrition

When you're older and lose excessive weight, you can develop protein energy malnutrition, which can set you up for anemia, hip fractures, infections, muscle weakness, and pressure ulcers. It actually compromises your immune system, which has already been negatively affected just by your getting older.

Triglycerides and Blood Cholesterol

Finally, losing fat weight causes *triglycerides* (stored in fat cells) to be released; they also come from excess fat in your liver. Too much pouring into your blood can raise the levels of the bad types of cholesterol, which are known to increase your risk for heart disease and stroke. When you lose body fat, you also potentially release a lifetime of accumulated toxins like PCBs and DDEs from insecticides, which are stored in the fat tissue.[18] This increase in circulating toxins could potentially cause nerve damage and may be the primary reason why significant weight loss in your later years can be detrimental. We don't usually talk about this with our patients, though, and we only mention this so you can be aware of it.

THE "JUST RIGHT" WEIGHT FOR SENIORS

When we say that carrying some extra weight may actually benefit you, we're generally talking about an overall minor amount, not extreme obesity (like on *The Biggest Loser*). *Modest* weight gain throughout your later years is what we mean. What counts as modest? About 10 pounds per decade, or 1 pound a year, depending on the size of your body frame and how muscular you are, adding up to an extra 10–15 pounds in your later years. The actual amounts of healthy weight gain will vary by individual, and most studies have shown that keeping the weight off in your middle years benefits your health far into your later life.[4]

Carrying Some Extra Fat Weight

What is the health impact of carrying a few extra pounds when you're older? A recent study found that being "overweight" (according to your body mass index, or BMI) is not associated with a higher risk of dying, at least not in over half a million US adults followed for only nine years, including study participants over 65.[19] A 21%–108% greater mortality risk was associated with being in the "obese" category with a BMI equal to or greater than 30. While BMI is not necessarily the best way to measure weight changes over time since it can't account for what percentage of your weight is fat and what's muscle and other things, these findings do support the notion that not all weight gain is bad as you get older, although gaining too much can be.

Losing Modest Amounts of Weight

That said, large clinical studies such as the US Diabetes Prevention Program have found that weight loss in middle age (in your 50s and 60s) lowers the risk of prediabetes progressing to type 2 diabetes and of other health problems.[20] That ongoing study also included regular physical activity and a focus on modest weight loss, and later follow-ups have shown that the people who started out at low fitness levels gained the most benefit when it came to diabetes prevention and keeping up their physical activity. Active individuals usually gain less fat weight and retain and gain more muscle, which may explain many of the benefits of regular activity for better long-term health.

Losing Weight the Right Way

If you do want to lose a few pounds, all diets have been shown to work in the short run as long as you're taking in fewer calories than your body needs. Even the type of diet (in terms of carbohydrate content and calorie count) that young people with type 1 diabetes follow to lose weight doesn't appear to matter.[21] It's best to avoid going on very low calorie diets since they invariably cause you to lose muscle mass along with fat and can leave you short on vital nutrients, vitamins, and minerals. It's also easy to regain the weight as soon as you're back to eating normally.

It's imperative to exercise regularly if you go on a diet in order to slow the loss of muscle. Try aerobic activities as well as resistance training.[22] Just expect your weight loss to be slower (at least on the bathroom scale) when you exercise while dieting since it's helping you retain more muscle, which contains a lot of water and fewer stored calories than body fat. And know that your body composition is changing for the better.

Preventing Weight Regain

The big challenge is keeping yourself from regaining any weight you lost while dieting. We've all been there and seen other people go through it as well. It's important that you make permanent lifestyle improvements that benefit your weight and your health concurrently. Staying physically active is one of the key changes that really help to prevent weight regain—even if that just means being more mindful about moving as much as possible each day. It's also important to continue down the path of better eating and be conscious about your food choices and the size of your portions. Gaining weight, or regaining what you've lost, is mostly easily prevented with a "small changes" approach, and that is easier to maintain over a lifetime.[23]

Taming Visceral Fat

We've mentioned it repeatedly in this step already, but *visceral* fat can be defined as belly fat located deep within your abdominal cavity that surrounds organs like your liver and pancreas and areas like your stomach and intestines. The other main type of fat in your body is stored directly under the surface of your skin (*subcutaneous*)—your "pinch an inch" fat.

How can you get rid of the type of deep abdominal fat that's making you unhealthier? Focus on making better lifestyle choices, the same you'd use to manage your body weight. Try some of the following:

- **Exercise training:** Any type of exercise training has been shown in studies to reduce visceral fat and insulin resistance—two wins! Even adding some faster intervals into your normal exercise routines can help you lose it faster.
- **Healthier eating:** Keep following your heathy diet as well, and try to limit your intake of trans fat, refined carbohydrates and sugar, and highly processed foods. Try out some prebiotics and probiotics.
- **Occasional fasting:** In some studies, intermittent fasting (going through periods of eating and not eating) can help lower visceral fat—but check with your doctor before doing

that to ensure none of your meds or their doses need adjusting
to go through the fasting periods safely.

- **Sleeping better:** Try to get enough sleep and good sleep.
  Getting too-little shut-eye or sleeping poorly can raise levels of
  the hormone cortisol, released when your body is under stress,
  and this can cause an excess of visceral fat in particular.
- **Reducing stress:** Feeling stressed or anxious can also raise
  your cortisol levels, so try to find ways to relax and turn off your
  fight-or-flight responses.
- **Drinking less alcohol:** Alcohol itself contains 7 calories per
  gram, and the average glass of wine or beer has 100 or more
  calories. Mixers used with hard liquors can contain a lot of extra
  calories and sugar as well, potentially all adding to your visceral
  fat stores. Try limiting your alcohol intake to no more than the
  recommended levels (one drink daily for women, two for men).

ASSESSING YOUR BODY WEIGHT AND FATNESS

When it comes to your body, there are various ways to assess its size
and the impact it may be having on your health. Historically, you just
weighed yourself on a bathroom scale, but even those numbers can
be misleading. In assessing population health, researchers and clinicians have used the BMI value, along with others that are gaining
traction like waist circumference. It's also possible to directly measure your body fat with special tools.

Scale Weight

Measuring body weight on a scale is commonplace. It's okay to use for
general trends, but many things can affect the exact number, including
the time of day, what you're wearing, whether you're dehydrated, and

more. To use it for trending purposes, it's best to weigh yourself each time under similar circumstances—such as first thing in the morning before you take a shower with the same clothing on each time.

It's not unusual for your weight to vary by a few pounds or more from day to day or even within a single day. Exercising outdoors and excessive sweating can make you lose pounds that you will quickly replace once you rehydrate. Eating a large meal or excess salt intake can bump your weight up (temporarily). That's why it's best to stick to one time of day and control as many of these factors as possible if you really want to know whether your body weight has changed in a meaningful way. We usually advise people to follow their bodily changes using other methods in addition to scale weight.

Body Mass Index

Many doctors record your weight and height and then calculate your body mass index (BMI) when you go in for an office visit. A BMI of 30 or more is considered obesity, and you likely have a higher level of intra-abdominal visceral fat at that number and above. They calculate your BMI because it's quick and easy, but it can be very misleading. Both your body weight on a scale and your BMI follow a U-shaped curve for your risk of dying, meaning that you're better off if your BMI is neither very low nor very high (both of which increase your health risk).

BMI doesn't account for your body fat percentage and variations in disease risk based on BMI alone in various groups of people. There's also an ongoing discussion about which BMI levels lower your health risks, and new guidelines for normal ranges when using BMI for health screenings have been issued for different populations (such as people with an Asian genetic makeup) because some develop type 2 diabetes at much lower BMIs than other groups.[24] A newer "body roundness index" (BRI) including height and waist measures and not weight may replace BMI at some point.

In any case, a "healthy" BMI range rises slightly as you age, from an average BMI of 21.4 when you are 20–29 years old up to 26.6 for 60–69-year-olds. This is not reflected in most BMI and health-risk tables, which are more suited to younger people. In a 2016 study, nearly 50% of all participants who fell into an "overweight" category and almost 30% considered to have obesity were metabolically healthy, while over 30% in a "normal" range were found to be unhealthy.[25] Even people who were metabolically healthy and obese over several decades still had a higher risk of heart and other cardiovascular diseases.[26]

The American Medical Association recently issued a policy advising doctors not to simply determine a healthy weight with BMI; they advised using waist circumference, fat distribution in the body, and genetic factors to assess health. In that same study, people with a higher waist measurement but the same BMI had a higher risk of death overall, reflecting the negative impact of having more fat stored around your middle. Having obesity—instead of just being overweight—by BMI standards increases the risk of dying whether people are young or old.[19]

You can access any online BMI calculator to put in your height and weight and find out your number, such as the one found on the National Institutes of Health website at https://www.nhlbi.nih.gov/health/educational/lose_wt/BMI/bmicalc.htm (box 6.4). Keep in mind that BMI is a really poor measure of relative amounts of fat and muscle, and very muscular individuals can end up "overweight" by BMI standards. As you age, you're also losing some height, which raises your BMI. BMI also fails to account for any losses in your bone mineral density as you get older.

Waist Circumference

While a favored measurement to determine the risk of type 2 diabetes and other health issues has traditionally been the waist-to-hip

> **Box 6.4**
> **Determining BMI and Visceral Fat Risk**
>
> **BMI:** Divide your weight by the square of your height (weight over height^2). Take your weight in pounds and your height in inches (squared) and multiply by 705. For instance, if you weigh 165 pounds and are 5 feet 9 inches tall, your BMI is the following: $165/(69 \times 69) = 165/4761 = 0.035 \times 705 = 24.6$.
>
> **Waist Circumference:** Wrap a tape measure around your waist just above your hip bones. For women, 35 inches or more means you're at risk for health problems related to central adiposity (visceral fat). For men, the number is 40 inches or greater.

ratio, things have shifted a bit. Waist circumference alone (the distance around your waist in inches or centimeters), an indicator of visceral fat, may be an accurate predictor. Men whose waists are 37.9–39.8 inches, for example, have a fivefold greater risk of diabetes than men whose waists are 29–34 inches. Women's waists should be less than 34.7 inches to lower their diabetes and heart disease risk, but their waists tend to start increasing after menopause.

Why does waist size matter—other than trying to fit into your pants? Your waist is indicative of where you store any extra fat. Obesity can be abdominal (central) or peripheral (lower body), also known as *android* and *gynoid* obesity, respectively. When you store fat around your abdomen, neck, shoulder, and arms, you have more of an "apple" shape, often associated with males. Much of this extra fat is actually stored within the abdomen, in and around your organs and even in your liver, pancreas, and heart—places where fat can negatively affect your metabolism and your health. This more metabolically active visceral fat may be easier to gain and lose, but it's also commonly associated with insulin resistance, type 2 diabetes, high blood pressure, heart disease, and even cognitive decline and dementia (see the next section for ways to lose visceral fat).

A recent study has found that having more visceral fat and fat in your pancreas is associated with a greater risk of developing type 2 diabetes, so where you have extra fat really does matter.[27] This central obesity is far more dangerous to your long-term health than being a "pear," which is more common in females and involves carrying extra weight in your hips, thighs, and buttocks. Anyone can end up with muscles riddled with fat like a steak, which is an unhealthy condition as well. Unfortunately, you can't control where you store fat (that's up to your genes), but you can help manage the total amount with your lifestyle choices, and exercising is a proven way to decrease unhealthy fat storage.[28]

Body Composition

Measuring your body fat percentage is possible with some special tools that can determine what's fat in your body and what's everything else (water, muscle, bone, internal organs, etc.). This matters because two people of the same weight can have entirely different amounts of muscle and fat and fall into various health ratings based on those differences.

In Dr. Colberg's exercise physiology courses, she teaches all the methods used to test body composition, but most aren't easily accessible, such as body fat calipers, underwater weighing, and dual-energy X-ray absorptiometry (DEXA) scans. The main one you may be able to measure on your own is *bioelectrical impedance analysis,* using one of those newfangled bathroom scales with the metal electrodes that you stand on. This method of testing is notoriously inaccurate, though, and affected by things such as room temperature, how cold your feet are, and when you last ate. It may be able to give you trends; for instance, if your body fat measure goes up from one day to the next, you may be dehydrated (since body water falls into the not-fat category). If you have a professional scan to measure your bone density, it may be possible to get the results of your body composition at the same time since they both use a DEXA scanner.

PREVENTING UNHEALTHY WEIGHT LOSS AS YOU AGE

For most of your adult life, you likely focused on not gaining too much weight, but losing too much after you're past 70 can be more of a concern. As mentioned, it can often be a sign of failing health, and in studies it has certainly been associated with hip fractures, an increased risk of dying from all causes, and having to go into a nursing home.

Let's talk about why weight loss is more common after 60 and what you can do about it. A list of possible reversible causes of weight loss can easily be remembered using the acronym MEALS-ON-WHEELS (box 6.5). We'll discuss a select few of them in more detail as well.

Diminished Appetite and Muscle Loss

One of the main causes of weight loss in your later years is simply eating less, which can be driven by many things, including being less active. Many people experience a decreased appetite when they're older, in part because their sense of taste and smell have diminished with age, and they no longer enjoy foods like they used to. Others have recently lost these senses from having COVID-19, and some have never regained them. Having less of an appetite isn't an issue unless it's leading you to lose a lot of weight. If your weight is stable even with a lesser appetite, then it's not a problem. If you are losing weight,

Box 6.5
Reversible Causes of Weight Loss (MEALS-ON-WHEELS)

Medications

Emotions (e.g., depression)

Anorexia (nervosa or tardive), alcoholism, or abuse

Late-life paranoia

Swallowing disorders

Oral factors (like dentures and missing teeth)

No money or noscomial infections (illnesses acquired in a hospital, such as tuberculosis)

Wandering and other dementia-related behaviors

Hyperthyroidism, hyperparathyroidism, or poorly managed diabetes

Entry (digestive) problems or malabsorption

Eating problems or gallstones (*cholecystitis*)

Low-salt or low-cholesterol diet (unpalatable therapeutic diet)

Shopping or food preparation issues

try eating multiple small meals so that your stomach never feels overly full, and take in high-calorie supplements and snacks between meals.

A flagging appetite, if ignored, can lead to muscle wasting, or sarcopenia, mentioned earlier in this step. To live long and well, your goal should be to have as much healthy muscle as possible. Losing too much muscle tends to lead to frailty and early death. Many of the causes of a poor appetite that lead to muscle loss are reversible. Consider these tips to help with your eating:

- **Take fewer or change your medications:** A combination of multiple meds can lower your appetite. Talk with your doctor about trying others, lowering some of your doses, or substituting for those with less of an impact on your appetite. (This is particularly true when you're using incretin mimetics for your diabetes management, as they may suppress your appetite or cause early stomach fullness.)

- **Manage your stomach and intestinal health:** Chronic pain can make it more difficult to eat, as can nausea, acid reflux, chronic diarrhea or frequent constipation, stomach fullness when eating, or a diabetes-related complication called *gastroparesis*, which delays your stomach emptying. Talk to your doctor about what you can do to improve your gastrointestinal health, and consider prebiotics or probiotics as well.
- **Fix your dentures or your teeth:** Problems with your dentures or missing and unstable teeth can make it harder to eat and cause you to ultimately eat less. Try having them affixed better, getting dental work to replace some teeth (like implants), or preparing foods differently to make them easier to chew.
- **Address your blues:** Feeling depressed can cause you to lose your appetite and should be treated sooner rather than later for that reason.

Cytokines and Muscle Wasting

We talked about cytokines when we addressed inflammation in step 2 and earlier in this step. An excessive release of cytokines has an inflammatory effect. Cytokines also have less obvious effects, such as leaching calcium out of your bones, pulling proteins out of muscle, decreasing red blood cells, interfering with memory, causing anemia, and generally making you feel sick. Two cytokines, interleukin-6 (IL-6) and tumor necrosis factor alpha (TNF-alpha), tend to increase during the normal aging process and lead to a loss of muscle fibers as well. Elevated levels of IL-6 increase your risk of disability.[29] If you have rheumatoid arthritis, lung problems, or heart failure,

192 • AGING WELL WITH DIABETES

increased levels of both IL-6 and TNF-alpha can lead to muscle wasting and reduced strength.[30] Excess cytokines likely play a key role in the muscle wasting that accompanies aging.

Treatments for Muscle Loss

Although you can't completely prevent some sarcopenia from occurring, you can combat your loss of muscle mass with resistance training, creatine supplements, testosterone, and appetite enhancers. Since your muscles are constantly being broken down and rebuilt, anything affecting that directly can alter the balance between increases in size and loss of mass.

Resistance training: For a full discussion of resistance training, refer back to step 3. While you may not be able to regain all the muscle you lost, you can at least slow the rate of additional losses and possibly regain some.

Creatine: Some people have used creatine supplements, along with resistance training, to try to preserve muscle and gain a little. It has been a popular supplement among the power-lifting and weight-training younger crowd but also has measurable effects when combined with exercise training. In one study, adults aged 57–70 who supplemented with creatine for 7 to 52 days while engaging in regular resistance training experienced a significant increase in their muscle mass, and another showed a positive impact on blood glucose levels in those with type 2 diabetes.[31,32]

Testosterone: An anabolic steroid that stimulates muscle growth and repair, testosterone is higher in males than females but declines with advancing age in everyone. It can be prescribed to combat excessive muscle loss with aging but only if your blood levels are very low. You generally can't prevent or reverse all age-related declines in muscle with testosterone, but you may be able to slow them if low testosterone is the cause.

Appetite-boosters: Another treatment involves the use of appetite-boosting drugs—but only if your reduced appetite is causing you to lose muscle. Some people with AIDS have been prescribed dronabinol, a medication made from an active cannabis extract of marijuana, a recreational drug known for causing the "munchies" in its users. Since many states have legalized medical and/or recreational marijuana, it may be available without a prescription. But always make sure your doctor knows you're taking it so they can recognize any interactions with your prescribed meds.

Another prescribed drug that enhances appetite is Megace (and Megace ES), a progestational steroid that cuts down on cytokine release while enhancing appetite and promoting weight gain. Another option is oxandrolone, an oral steroid that helps people gain weight following surgery, trauma, or chronic infection.

Although dronabinol, megestrol acetate, abd oxandrolone, and dronabinol are the only FDA-approved drugs used as appetite stimulants, others enhance appetite and have been prescribed off-label for that purpose. These include some antidepressants (e.g., mirtazapine) and corticosteroids (like prednisone and dexamethasone), but watch out for the glucose-raising impact of the latter and their other potential side effects.

In this step, we've talked about the dangers of gaining too much fat (especially when you're packing the extra fat abdominally) or losing too much muscle. Both are associated with health problems and an increased risk of dying early. Regular exercise is the best strategy for fat weight loss and weight maintenance, but to reverse your loss of appetite if it's causing muscle wasting, you may need to seek medical help. In the end, Dr. Munshi always tells her patients to concentrate on the process and not on the results. If you eat healthy and exercise, you won't need to focus on your actual weight the same way.

CHAPTER SEVEN

Step 7: Rev Up Your Brain Power

Did you know that one of the biggest problems associated with aging with diabetes is a loss of brain function over time? Brain health becomes even more critical to address since cognitive impairment and dementia are much more common when you're older and can be accelerated by having diabetes. Figuring out and managing your diabetes regimen and your overall health can be much more challenging with less brain power. But you can rev it up with lifestyle changes such as more physical activity and medication adjustments, and simplify your regimen to make it easier to follow. If you start feeling depressed, anxious, or emotionally distressed, there are lifestyle changes you can make to improve your mental health as well (box 7.1).

Humans' ability to think and reason allows us to interact with others in ways that other animal species can't. It's a precious gift to have cognitive skills that allow us to learn new things and adapt to the changing world around us. You may find, though, that you're losing some of that ability as you age. Learning can definitely slow at older ages, as can being able to reason things out. Many older individuals end up suffering from cognitive impairment and dementia, which

> **Box 7.1**
>
> **Step 7: Rev Up Your Brain Power**
>
> - What's old
>   - Expecting your memory to fail and your mind to lose its sharpness as you age—and assuming there is nothing you can do about it
> - What's new
>   - Knowing that brain health and body health are interlinked and that working on one benefits the other
> - What you should be doing
>   - Taking action to improve your brain power (and your body) health

can dramatically reduce your quality of life and cause family and friends to "lose" the "you" they have known.

A declining memory or other changes in your mental or emotional health can take its toll on you and your family members. Dementia is the most common illness to affect the older brain, and Alzheimer's disease occurs more frequently in people with diabetes.[1] But you can also suffer from depression, anxiety, and other mental and emotional disorders that can negatively affect your life and exacerbate feelings of memory loss (box 7.2). There is help for many emotional conditions, however, and some level of memory loss is considered normal. The trick is to know the difference and to prepare for and prevent unnecessary losses.

MANAGE YOUR BRAIN HEALTH

First, let's talk about your brain, ability to learn, and memory. We've all relied on our learning and memory abilities to manage our adult

196 • AGING WELL WITH DIABETES

> **Box 7.2**
> **Insight from Dr. Munshi**
>
> I see two 80-year-old patients with diabetes with similar medications and similar blood glucose management. One says, "I am the luckiest person in the world. I have the best doctors, a happy family, good health, and, hey, I wake up every day to live another day." Another one says, "My life is miserable. I have to go see doctors every day, my family never calls me, and I wonder why I am alive."
>
> These two very different ways of thinking make a world of difference when it comes to how people care for their chronic diseases and how they feel about them.
>
> We did a research study on 165 older adults with type 1 diabetes. These people took care of their diabetes when technology was nonexistent, insulin needles were thick, and urine testing was the only way to test glucose at all—and yet I have never seen people with a more positive attitude. Did that attitude make them survivors? Or is that how they became survivors? I can only suggest that, regardless of which came first, it will benefit you to follow that same path when choosing how to feel about your life.

lives and to take care of ourselves and others (including kids, grandkids, aging relatives, friends, and pets). You probably want to know what causes memory loss and how much is normal to forget. You may also want to know what causes dementia and how you can lower the risk of it and Alzheimer's disease. These are all important topics to understand and know more about as you age.

What Role Do Neurotransmitters Play in Brain Health?

Your brain relies on neural connections and *neurotransmitters*, which are chemical messengers that—in the case of your brain specifically—carry messages from one nerve cell to the next. Examples include glutamate, GABA, dopamine, serotonin, acetylcholine, and endorphins, some of which are excitatory and others inhibitory. Many of these are involved in the creation and transmission of your thoughts, memory, learning, and feelings. One of the most excitatory brain neurotransmitters is glutamate, which is involved in all of these and is often associated with Alzheimer's disease, dementia, Parkinson's disease, and seizures when levels become unbalanced or deficient.[2]

What Causes Your Neurotransmitters to Malfunction?

A number of scenarios are possible when it comes to malfunctioning brain neurotransmission. It's possible to produce too much or too little of a brain neurotransmitter, with varying results based on which one is affected. The brain neurons that usually receive a signal from a specific neurotransmitter may also have faulty receptors, blocking or slowing any communication from an otherwise normal messenger. In some cases, neurotransmitters are released and then stay around too long or get reabsorbed too quickly, creating issues.

Enzymes in the brain may limit the number of neurotransmitters reaching their target cell, or you may have problems with other parts of your brain or medications that have an impact on neurotransmitters.

Here are some examples of neurotransmitter malfunctions and results:

- **Acetylcholine:** a lack can lead to the memory loss typical with Alzheimer's disease.
- **Serotonin:** excesses have been associated with autism spectrum disorders.
- **Glutamate and GABA:** the increased activity of glutamate or decreased activity of GABA may cause sudden, high-frequency firing of brain neurons and seizures.
- **Norepinephrine and dopamine:** the excessive activity of these and abnormal glutamate transmission may lead to mania in bipolar disorder.

What Is Memory and How Do We Lose It?

Things that you experience or learn go first into what's called your *short-term memory*. That's when you remember things for minutes to days after learning them. Items can also be moved over into your *long-term memory*, where they can be kept for months, years, and decades. Unlike sensory and short-term memory, which are limited and decay rapidly, long-term memory can store unlimited amounts of information for an indefinite period of time. You can start losing either one of these types of memory without the other type being affected, and what you're losing may indicate the specific brain issues affecting you.

Losing some of your ability to learn new things happens to almost everyone who lives long enough, but it is more dependent on your short-term memory. Your long-term memory, on the other hand, includes remembering events and facts and how to complete tasks, such as tying your shoes (assuming you already knew how), making toast, and finding your way home (something that should be second nature to most people). Having and retaining these long-term abilities can be critical for living independently as you get on in years.

Experiencing a slower rate of learning and memorizing facts is normal, but losing either your short-term or your long-term memory should not occur due to aging alone. You may become more forgetful, but you should still be able to do most of your usual activities and remember critical events and people (like your spouse or partner, children and grandkids, close friends, and more). You might forget the name of a book you read or a movie you recently saw, but you shouldn't forget that you read or saw it. Also, forgetting who your close relatives and friends are is definitely concerning.

Most older adults who complain about forgetting things don't have Alzheimer's disease, or even dementia. They are more likely experiencing normal levels of forgetfulness or have a mental or medical cause for not remembering, such as mild cognitive impairment, depression, stress, anxiety, fatigue, lack of sleep, or a prior head trauma that's affecting their memory. Some of these symptoms result from simply trying to do too many things at once, as we almost all are in this modern world where we're constantly multitasking. Deficiencies in vitamin B_{12} and folate intake can also increase memory issues, so keep that in mind if you take metformin since it can cause the loss of some of the B vitamins (which can be restored with supplements).[3]

Having diabetes itself can have an impact on your memory under certain circumstances. Not remembering things that happened while your blood glucose was too low can be normal—your brain needs glucose to function optimally and form memories. On the flip side, blood glucose levels higher than 200 mg/dL have also been shown to interfere with normal learning and memory, as can triglyceride (blood fat) levels above 150 mg/dL.[4]

So how can you know whether your memory loss is truly concerning? Not all memory issues are permanent; many are actually reversible (box 7.3). As the retired geriatrician Dr. John Morley noted in another book on aging well, "Sometimes the 'cure' is incredibly simple, such as when medical students at Saint Louis University found that simply removing excess wax from the ears of nursing home residents improved their mental status more than most drugs."[5] All possible medical causes of memory loss should be considered and ruled out before you can be diagnosed with a more serious issue such as dementia or Alzheimer's disease.

As mentioned, some forgetfulness is normal, as is losing some of your ability to ride a bike, judge distances, and learn new facts. These are all part of age-related changes to your brain and neurotransmitter function. In fact, we all have our own personal quirks. For example, Dr. Munshi is really bad at remembering names, and she has had this

Box 7.3
Reversible Causes of Memory Loss (DEMENTIA)

- **D**—drugs: certain antidepressants, antipsychotics, digoxin, and others
- **E**—emotions: depression, anxiety, stress, and trauma
- **M**—metabolic disorders: low thyroid function, poorly managed blood glucose levels, low vitamin B_{12} levels
- **E**—eyes and ears: hearing and vision issues
- **N**—normal pressure hydrocephalus: a rare disorder curable by inserting a shunt into the brain's ventricles to drain excess cerebrospinal fluid
- **T**—tumors and other space-occupying lesions: bleeding into the head following trauma, benign or malignant brain tumors
- **I**—infections: AIDS, Lyme disease, COVID-19, syphilis, and many others
- **A**—anemia: low hemoglobin levels, fewer red blood cells

trait since she was very young. She's really good at remembering stories, however. So she may not remember your name, but once she sees you, she remembers well what has happened to you and your life story. Many healthy older adults retain their overall intellectual performance into their 80s and beyond, including items like language ability, sensory and immediate memory, and problem-solving skills. And most of them are physically active, which helps improve your memory and cognitive skills.

Simply moving your body—that is, exercising—may improve your memory. Think how important memory was to early man when it came to hunting for food for survival. Modern man still thinks better and remembers more when active (box 7.4).

You may also experience some cognitive impairment related to physiological or psychological conditions, due not only to reversible

Box 7.4
How Does Exercise Improve Your Memory?

Exercise enhances your memory in two ways. First, your heart is pumping more and perfusing your brain with nutrient-rich blood when you're active. This results in better neural connections and memory formation, along with generally better cardiovascular health over the long haul.

Second, exercising can have a direct impact on growth factors in the brain that nourish its cells. These growth factors are essential for the brain to repair small injuries to remain healthy and functional. Both brain-derived neurotrophic factor and nerve growth factor increase significantly during exercise, which helps with memory. In short, being physically active helps your brain repair itself so you can learn and form memories more effectively.

causes like depression but also from more serious issues like stroke, Alzheimer's disease, Parkinson's disease, certain tumors, cardiovascular problems, schizophrenia, and severe anxiety. Ask your doctor to check whether your cognitive changes result from a reversible condition or a more permanent one.

Is It Mild Cognitive Impairment or Dementia?

If you're experiencing small alterations in your ability to think—and your blood glucose is normal—you may have *mild cognitive impairment*. What that means is that you may be experiencing some issues with your memory, speaking, or decision-making at this stage—which can happen with aging—but you haven't reached the point of actually having dementia. You may feel like your memory is slipping but still be able to function mostly normally. Mild impairment progresses to some form of dementia within five years in about half of people with noticeable cognitive changes.

Approximately half of all adults develop some level of *dementia* if they live long enough—by which we mean memory loss plus deficits

202 • AGING WELL WITH DIABETES

in one or more of your cognitive abilities. To be diagnosed with dementia, you must have lost some of your ability to perform normal tasks like handle your finances or take your medications. Dementia has many potential causes, such as high blood pressure resulting in vascular changes that reduce blood flow to the brain (common in diabetes).[1] Alzheimer's disease is the most common form of dementia, accounting for as much as 70% of cases. You can have other forms as well, such as vascular dementia (related to reduced blood flow to the brain), Lewy body dementia (caused by protein deposits inside of nerve cells where they shouldn't be), and frontotemporal dementia (related to brain frontal lobe degeneration, which can be caused by a number of diseases; table 7.1).

Few prescription medications are available to effectively manage dementia, so the best thing you can do is treat any reversible causes

Table 7.1. Characteristics of Alzheimer's Disease, Vascular Dementia, and Depression

	Alzheimer's disease	Vascular dementia	Depression
Onset	Gradual and subtle	Abrupt	Gradual and variable
Progression	Slow progression with fluctuations	Stepwise	Progressive with remissions
Features	Deficits in at least two cognitive areas, altered behavior, illusions, delusions, hallucinations, muscle rigidity, seizures (late stages of disease), altered gait	Evidence of vascular disease but only intermittent defects in cognition	Subjective complaints, sad, poor motivation
Neuroimaging changes	Loss of volume of hippocampus	Multiple vascular lesions	None

of memory loss that may be contributing. If you have vascular problems—which are common in people with diabetes—treating those to enhance blood flow to the brain can improve symptoms.[6]

When it comes to managing diabetes, any form of dementia can cause issues with self-care and handling blood glucose levels. Dr. Munshi has noticed that older adults with diabetes have more difficulty with problem-solving, planning, and organizing, not necessarily just memory issues. They also often have difficulty being attentive, starting a new behavior, or stopping an old one. Diabetes care involves these skills and behaviors, so managing it can become very challenging, especially if people have trouble monitoring blood glucose, taking medication, following diet plans, and obtaining more physical activity. Dr. Munshi knows firsthand that when her older adult patients have any level of cognitive dysfunction, she must be mindful of their level of cognitive decline and refrain from giving them any tasks that go beyond their capabilities.

Is It Alzheimer's Disease?

Although it can be devastating when Alzheimer's disease occurs, only about 1 in 13 people aged 65–84 and 1 in 3 people aged 85 and older are living with Alzheimer's.[7] Most people now agree that there is no single cause of Alzheimer's and that it's more likely the result of genetics, environmental influences, health conditions, and even lifestyle factors, such as diet and physical activity levels. Some of these contributing factors, nevertheless, are interrelated. For instance, blocking the overproduction of beta-amyloid protein buildup (one contributing cause) in the brain reduces oxidative damage, another potential contributor to disease onset. Increased levels of a brain protein called tau can cause the development of neurofibrillary tangles (as seen in Alzheimer's) and dementia without a lot of beta-amyloid present.[8] In some cases, supplementing with alpha-lipoic acid to reduce oxidative damage leads to improved memory.

Systemic inflammation is also a contributing factor to this disease onset. We spent all of step 2 talking about ways to manage and reduce inflammation. Elevated levels of insulin, like most people have when they're insulin resistant, add to inflammation. The small amount of insulin usually found in the brain disappears early in the course of Alzheimer's disease, and the lack of it contributes to a decreased clearance of beta-amyloid. These associations may explain why the risk of Alzheimer's disease is higher for anyone with diabetes. Some have found that using insulin sensitizers can improve your mental status and memory. Now is when you should refer back to steps 3 and 4 to help you make the lifestyle changes that may keep you from ever developing Alzheimer's, even if you do have diabetes. A healthy cardiovascular system is also vitally important for brain health. The more risk factors you have for cardiovascular diseases, including smoking, high blood pressure, insulin resistance, and physical inactivity, the more likely you are to develop Alzheimer's disease. Use your lifestyle choices to keep your brain healthy and prevent mental declines.[9,10]

MANAGING DEPRESSION

Feeling a little bit sad or blue on occasion can be normal, but pervasive and overwhelming sadness, especially without a cause, such as a death in the family, can erode your ability to function, often leading to suicidal thoughts and actions. In a study at the Joslin Geriatric Diabetes Clinic, Dr. Munshi noted that approximately one-third of her patients had symptoms of depression. People with diabetes are about twice as likely to be depressed as those without diabetes, and the rate increases with age.[11]

What Causes Depression?

While multiple factors can contribute to depression, the demands of self-care for those with diabetes may be a contributory cause for many people. Dr. Munshi knows that both depression and dementia have a bidirectional relationship with diabetes. Keeping their depression under control can help people cope with their diabetes. You need to manage your depression without setting yourself up for failure by setting unrealistic goals. Your goals shouldn't necessarily depend on your age but rather on your other medical issues, if any. What is your cognitive, functional, and emotional status (box 7.5)? What are you being treated with? Recent studies have shown that if we treat depression successfully, people can improve blood glucose management.[12] It's important for other aspects of your mental and emotional health to develop a regimen that fits your ability to care for yourself.

Box 7.5
Look Out for These Signs of Cognitive Changes or Depression

- Your blood glucose levels are suddenly worse even though you've been doing fairly well with them on your own (related to cognitive changes or depression).
- You may have subtle changes in your mental status, such as being more forgetful about monitoring your blood glucose or taking medications, making mistakes in doses of insulin, or even forgetting to eat a meal (related to either).
- You may be having trouble coping with multiple medical conditions or medications and appear stressed or overwhelmed by them (related to either).
- You may gradually become less socially active or engaged with others, drop activities that you used to enjoy, or show other signs of depression, such as sadness or hopelessness or isolation from your friends and family (related to depression).

Depression can also arise from experiencing diabetes-related and other health complications, so you should seek to prevent those whenever possible. Some approaches to managing depression include therapy (especially cognitive behavioral, or CBT, therapy) and medications to help manage your moods. Mood regulation is essential to overall well-being, so paying attention to emotional and mental disruptions is important. Your goal as you age is to remain functional and independent so you can live your life the way you want to. Quality of life is important and needs to be considered in the context of all these other factors, and it can help you avoid feeling depressed about having to manage diabetes. In that case, you may take better care of yourself and it's self-fulfilling.

Even though life can be challenging at any age, major depression occurs more commonly in young women than in older ones.[13] As you get older, you learn more coping skills to deal with disease and adversity. The older you get, however, the more likely you are to have health issues, which may lead you to develop an intermediate version of sadness known as dysphoria. If you do become depressed when you're older, your depression may go unrecognized and untreated, as many health professionals overlook its signs and symptoms. You may therefore have to steer the ship to better mental health, asking for help when you think you need it.

Health issues like diabetes, stroke, cancer, Parkinson's disease, and many hormonal disorders are more likely to lead to depressive feelings. If you're depressed and have a heart attack, you're more likely to have another cardiac event within a year.[14] Abnormal levels of the neurotransmitters serotonin and norepinephrine are the biggest contributors to feelings of depression, while *corticotrophic releasing factor* leads more to physical signs, such as weight loss, disturbed sleep, constipation, erectile dysfunction, and decreased libido. It elevates your cortisol levels, which can make your blood glucose management more difficult, not to mention contributes to faster bone thinning. These are just some additional reasons why it's so important to seek treatment for depression when you're older and must contend with diabetes.

How Can Depression Be Treated?

Talk therapy (seeing a therapist) is the first line of treatment for depression. People's propensity to seek out such care on their own varies with their views on psychotherapy and cultural norms. For instance, among members of the Black community, systemic racism over decades has made them more wary of seeking psychological treatment, with many preferring to turn to their religion or church communities for support.[15]

Many prescription medications are available to treat depression, including *tricyclics*, which alter norepinephrine function, and *selective serotonin reuptake inhibitors* (SSRIs), which maintain higher levels of the feel-good hormone serotonin in the brain and more effectively treat severe depression. Like any medication, these may have some potentially unpleasant side effects, but if your doctor prescribes one, it is safe to take for many years without major side effects if you are tolerating it. Think about these medications for your brain as you would think about any for your heart or diabetes. They can improve all those hormonal and chemical imbalances and have you feeling and taking care of your body better. In addition, some people seek out herbal remedies, such as Saint John's wort, which has been shown to work on mild to moderate depression.[16]

As for other potential treatments, a Harvard University study looked at mental health factors in older adults (over 50) and reported a number of them that led people to be "happy-well" instead of "sad-sick" well into their later years.[17] For instance, those who fared better were more skilled at dealing with adversity, were in a

208 • AGING WELL WITH DIABETES

stable marriage, exercised, refrained from smoking, drank alcohol only moderately, and stayed closer to a normal body weight. Not surprising to anyone who has studied exercise like Dr. Colberg or Dr. Munshi, who practices what she preaches, the study also reported that regular exercise, especially resistance exercise, decreased symptoms of depression. It appears that being active may be one of the best treatments for depression out there, and it has mostly positive side effects.

FIND OTHER WAYS TO STAY MENTALLY HEALTHY

We mentioned how cultural nuances and a sense of community may dictate how some people cope with their mental health issues. It's important to include in our discussion the role that spirituality and organized religion can play in aging well. In general, both can improve your psychological outlook on your life but may have minimal impact on your physical health. Their main role is to act as coping mechanisms by giving people access to other outlets for emotional support. Many people pray during times of physical or mental stress, and it helps many deal with disability, illness, and the end of life. No matter how old you are, you're likely still trying to find things to do, ways to express yourself, and meaning in your life. Practicing religion or serving others in various ways may bring you deep personal satisfaction, comfort, and peace and help you to age more successfully. People who are part of religious communities generally live longer and function better but don't necessarily become more religious as they age.

How Can You Bring Spirituality into Your Life?

We brought this whole section in from another book on aging (in general) that Dr. Colberg wrote with Dr. Morley back in 2007 called

The Science of Staying Young.[5] It all still applies to anyone with diabetes and other chronic illnesses, and it continues to be a vitally important topic.

Spiritual awakening is a journey, and you may feel the call to embark on a spiritual path after going through a difficult time or when certain parts of your life are no longer flowing as smoothly as they once did. Sharing your unique, personal experiences, even if they are outside of traditional realms, can increase your feelings of spirituality. Talking about your dreams, daydreams, near-death experiences, visions, hallucinations, and more serves as a positive outlet for your emotions.

Similarly, feelings of hope are associated with longer survival. Hope may be used as a means of coping with aging because of its ability to improve your expectations for the future, motivate you to take action, or give you the means of fulfilling your goals. Religious and spiritual activity can even help you recover faster from illness or injury.

Finally, creating legacies is another very constructive approach to bringing meaning and spirituality into your life. They may be expressed as written or taped memoirs, photograph collections, memory gardens, family histories or genealogies, and autobiographies or life histories. For some, making trips to family homes or pilgrimages to locations of spiritual significance also increase positive feelings. For others, telephone calls, prayer circles, televised religious services, and sacred readings may offer hope and solace. As far as your physical health is concerned, though, making the effort to attend church services regularly is far better than simply watching tele-evangelists without moving from your home. People who go to churches, mosques, or synagogues tend to maintain their function longer than those

210 • AGING WELL WITH DIABETES

who don't. Just getting out of the house and getting some exercise may explain some of these differences.

How Else Can You Keep Your Mind Sharp?

When it comes to your mental fitness, it's the same as for your muscles: "Use it or lose it." You can't do resistance training for your mind, but you can practice mental exercises that can help you maintain and improve your memory and your overall cognition. Some of them focus on stimulating all your senses, while others employ logical thinking and reasoning abilities. Here are some daily mental exercises for you to try:

- Memorize any sort of list in the morning (with at least 5–10 items on it, such as a grocery list) and then try to recall as many of the items on your list as you can at the end of the day. If you're doing this exercise well, bump it up a level, and make it even more challenging using a greater number of items or more difficult ones.
- Memorize some phone numbers of your loved ones at the start of the day. At the end of the day, write down their names and numbers and do this again later in the week.
- Even if you're not good at art, pick an object to draw. Observe it first and then draw it from memory (this works your short-term memory). Do this activity every day for a week. At the end of the week, redraw all seven items from memory without looking to see what they were (this works your long-term memory).
- Wherever you go, make a mental note of how many people, pieces of furniture, artwork, or other objects are to your left, straight ahead, and to your right. If you've been there before, try to pick out any details that have changed since you were there last.

- When you go somewhere and then return home, try to draw a map or plan of the place you went to, and do this exercise every time you come back from somewhere new.
- Find a sentence in something you are reading, make a note of the words in that sentence, and try to make other sentences using those words in a different order, or try substituting in new words in several places.
- Play challenging games—be they board games or online—and use your mental acuity to play them well. Good ones to try are chess, checkers, bridge, Othello, and others, as long as they tax your mind. Try different games. (Dr. Colberg's parents have played Scrabble almost every afternoon since the start of the pandemic, and that game changes each time you draw new letters.)
- Along those same lines, do daily crossword puzzles, anagrams, and other word or reasoning games. Even sudoku, Wordle, LinkedIn puzzle games, and other trendy ones will work.
- Find new interests, new activities, and new partners to play games with or to take part in other stimulating activities.
- Learn a new language, either on your own using online programs like Babbel, Duolingo, Memrise, Mango Languages, Mondly, and LearnaLanguage.com or by taking a class. Sign up for other courses that are challenging and fun.
- Listen to a program on TV or read the news, and afterward try to write down a summary of all the main points of it.
- When you see a word, take note of the first two letters and then try to think of as many others that begin with the same two letters as you can, or use the last two letters of the word and think of words ending with those.

- When eating a complex food, think about what you're tasting and smelling and identify its individual ingredients, including the subtle flavorings of its herbs and spices.
- Continue using your senses in other ways by using your sense of touch (and possibly smell) to identify various objects with your eyes closed.
- Do something different or new every day to make you think and reason, such as varying your route to figure out a different way to arrive at the same place.
- Do math problems in your head, such as adding, subtracting, multiplying, dividing, and figuring out percentages from decimals. Focus on trying to get better at those you find particularly challenging (e.g., adding fractions).
- Play video games by yourself or with your kids and grandkids (or even great-grandkids), particularly those that require quick responses.
- Be creative in coming up with new and different ways to exercise your mind on a daily basis.
- Read a lot of different types of things, including fiction and nonfiction, and try to remember the authors' names and the titles of what you read and recall those later.

What Counts as a Brain-Stimulating Exercise?

Brain-stimulating exercises include activities from computer-based puzzle games and reading to playing sports and talking to people. To be effective, you have to be an active participant in the activity—meaning that passively watching television or videos online doesn't work your brain as much.

Exercises that work your brain can be as simple as performing everyday tasks, but do them mindfully in that case, paying full attention to your activity. Other exercises are specifically targeted to be mental gymnastics for the brain, designed to enhance memory, cognition, and/or creativity. Simply trying to exercise your brain every day will help boost its function and the connectivity between its various regions. You may like some exercises and dislike others, so try a range and pick those you enjoy the most.

If you go online, you can now find myriad websites offering memory games of various types that may be fun to try. In addition to the activities listed, you may also get some mental benefits from meditating, visualizing, building jigsaw puzzles, socializing, increasing your vocabulary (a new word a day is a place to start), learning to play a musical instrument, and taking up new hobbies (including painting, knitting, dancing, woodworking, and many more).

One more guaranteed way to work your brain is by doing physical activity of almost any kind. Dancing can be particularly challenging because it requires thinking about your movements, keeping your balance, and often interacting with others. Tai chi and yoga are also good mentally stimulating activities.

Dr. Munshi started this step by talking about two patients of the same age with completely different mental outlooks about aging, the only conclusion being that having a positive outlook and good brain health makes a huge difference (see box 7.2). Similarly, more than a decade ago Dr. Colberg interviewed over 60 people who had been living for a long time with diabetes, many of them well over 50 years, and not one of them had any signs of dementia or significant memory loss.

A great example of their collective functioning was Gerald Cleveland, who participated in a research study that found him to be the mental equivalent of a 20-year-old, even after 91 years of being alive and three-quarters of a century with diabetes. He was always busy doing something, be it consulting with others about how to eat better to manage blood glucose levels or being in charge of committees in his retirement community, where he lived until the time of his passing at age 93 from old age. Another inspiring example of a person with long-standing diabetes was Dr. Robert J. Stewart, a retired podiatrist. He was setting world records in the Senior Olympics doing track-and-field events like the long jump and pole vault at the age of 96. No moss was collecting under his (very old) feet—and he lived to be almost 103 (he's also the one who put a tablespoon of milled flaxseed in his breakfast cereal every morning that we mentioned back in step 4).

All those long-term diabetes survivors leave us with no doubt that an active body and a busy life lead to the maintenance of a fully functioning mind. We therefore all need to think about making the treatment of major brain issues and mental health disorders a central part of aging successfully.

CHAPTER EIGHT

Step 8: Sleep Well, Rest, and Recuperate

Are you finding good sleep harder to come by these days? Unfortunately, both getting older and having diabetes can have an impact on how well you sleep and how quickly you recover from physical activity or time off from exercising. In addition, getting enough good sleep can be affected by nightly fluctuations in blood glucose. Improving your sleep, though, is important for overall health and wellness and even more important if you're handling a chronic condition like diabetes. It has been shown to help reduce stress, increase recovery from exercise, and improve mood. So let's get started on improving our sleep hygiene (box 8.1).

Lots of things can influence how well you sleep, and they only seems to get worse with age. Being able to sleep is crucial for physical and mental health, though, so it's vitally important to find ways to sleep better (box 8.2). Think of sleep time as the period when your body sweeps all the cobwebs out of your brain and sets things right for the next day. Relaxing during the day when you're awake is also a way of clearing your mind. Recuperating from being active is extremely important to overall wellness.

AGING WELL WITH DIABETES

Box 8.1

Step 8: Sleep Well, Rest, and Recuperate

- What's old
  - Not sleeping well and feeling fatigued, run down, stressed out, and less optimistic about life
- What's new
  - Focusing on sleep hygiene, adequate rest, and recovery time from activities in order to manage stress, boost your immune system, and function at a higher level
- What you should be doing
  - Finding ways to rest, including power naps, restful activities, and mental rest and relaxation

---

Box 8.2

Insight from Dr. Munshi

It's difficult to talk about positive thinking, much less engage in it, unless you are well rested. I asked one of my patient if he sleeps well. He said, "Oh, that doesn't bother me. If I am not sleepy, in my mind I go and visit all these wonderful places in the world that I have traveled. I fall asleep happy." This advice actually helped me too.

Our brain corrects a lot of irregularities during sleep. For example, the improper folding of certain proteins that are harmful to our memory gets cleaned up while we are asleep. Finding ways to relax is also important to our mental and physical health and well-being.

UNDERSTANDING SLEEP AS YOU AGE

We all need to get enough shut-eye time. As mentioned, sleep plays a housekeeping role that consists of removing various toxins and other substances that build up in your brain while you're awake. Sleep affects a number of brain functions, first and foremost how your brain cells interact and communicate. You may think of sleep as a time of inactivity, but both your brain and your body remain quite active while you are asleep. You go through sleep cycles with and without rapid eye movement, and you usually shift and move your body around on a regular basis. Your dreams are not continuous—although they may feel that ways sometimes—but rather only occur during certain sleep cycles.

Sleep Stages and Their Bodily Impacts

Let's take a minute and review what your brain goes through when you're sleeping. What's most interesting about the stages is that you spend differing amounts of time in them as you get older, which can have an impact on your sleep quality.

Your nightly sojourn includes both *rapid eye movement* (REM) sleep and non-REM sleep (consisting of three stages). During each cycle, your brain has certain nerve activities and brain waves. When you first fall asleep, your non-REM cycles tend to be longer (even though you go through all three of them), and then you continue to cycle through both types (REM and non-REM) during the night, with increasingly longer, deeper REM periods typically occurring toward morning.

- **Sleep stage 1: non-REM.** This is when you go from being awake to falling asleep. It's short (a few minutes) and a period of light sleep. It's when your parasympathetic nervous system is helping to slow things down, including your heart rate, breathing frequency, and eye movements. Your muscles are relaxing as well, although you may experience some twitching during this stage. Your brain waves also slow (compared to their daytime levels).

- **Sleep stage 2: non-REM.** This stage helps you transition from light sleep to a deeper sleep state. Your heart rate slows further, your breathing rate falls, and your muscles continue to relax. In addition, your eyes stop moving, and your body starts to cool. In your brain, the waves continue but slow enough that you're only experiencing occasional, brief moments of electrical activity and neural transmissions. Each night, more time is spent in this sleep stage than any other.
- **Sleep stage 3: non-REM.** Now you're ready for some deep sleep, and that's what you get in this stage. Initially, you spend long intervals in stage 3, but their length shortens as the night progresses. Your heart rate, breathing, temperature, muscle movement, and brain waves are at their lowest levels during this period of sleep. You may be hard to rouse during this stage because of your deep state of sleep.
- **Sleep stage: REM.** You don't experience any REM sleep until you've been asleep for about an hour and a half. It's called rapid eye movement sleep because that's exactly what happens: your eyes move rapidly from side to side even though they're closed. Your brain waves are closer to your waking hours during this stage, and your breathing may increase and become less regular. You experience increases in your heart rate and blood pressure that approach your normal levels when awake. This is also when you do most of your dreaming. Some dreaming is possible during non-REM stages, but during REM sleep you're not likely to act out what is going on in your dreams—thankfully—because your arm and leg muscles don't move. You do solidify some of your memories during REM sleep and others during non-REM. One main impact of aging is that you spend less of your night in REM sleep.

What Sleeping Does for You

Most people should aim to sleep about eight hours a day, preferably at night, which means you spend about a third of your life asleep. Getting quality sleep and adequate amounts are vital to your physical and mental health. Interestingly, your muscles can recuperate during daytime hours as well, such as during sedentary times, but your brain needs you to be asleep to really carry out its maintenance and repair. You need to sleep in order to learn well. Sleeping allows your brain to form the neural connections it needs to create and store new memories. Without adequate sleep, your ability to concentrate will be lessened, and you may find it harder to respond quickly to events during waking hours.

What's more, in addition to your brain health your heart, lungs, and metabolism can all be affected by a lack of sleep, along with your mood, ability to fight off infections, stress management, and disease resistance. Chronically getting too little sleep or having poor-quality sleep can cause a number of health issues, including obesity, prediabetes, type 2 diabetes, hypertension, cardiovascular disease, and depression.[1,2]

How to Fall and Stay Asleep

By now, you've probably heard about *melatonin*, at least in the context of a supplement you can take to help minimize jet lag and sleep when you cross time zones. Melatonin is actually a hormone produced by a small area in the middle of your brain called the *pineal gland*. The main role we think of melatonin playing is helping you adjust your *circadian rhythm*, or your day-night internal clock. Sometimes called our "third eye," the pineal gland actually contains light-sensitive cells, which is why we're more likely to be awake during daytime hours when melatonin secretion is lowest and asleep when it's dark and our blood levels of melatonin peak.[3]

One problem with getting adequate sleep when you're older is that your pineal gland actually starts to calcify, and these changes lead to lower levels of melatonin in your blood. In addition to inducing sleep, this hormone is thought to enhance your immune system and act as a powerful antioxidant, making it a potential antiaging hormone. Dr. Colberg and her late research colleague, Dr. Aaron I. Vinik, looked at type 2 diabetes as partly resulting from a dysfunction of normal circadian rhythms, suggesting that adequate melatonin levels may be very important for your overall health.[4]

Does that mean that you should supplement with melatonin as you get older? Dr. Colberg did a study on taking such supplements (10 mg of melatonin 30 minutes before bedtime) in older individuals with type 2 diabetes, and subjects reported an easier time falling sleep and lower blood glucose levels in the morning (compared to when they took a placebo).[5] It may not help you stay asleep longer. But if your lack of sleep is making your blood glucose levels rise overnight, it may be worth a try.

Sleep Disorders and How to Correct Them

Getting adequate sleep can be a problem, as there are more than 100 different sleep disorders. Some of them are common and are likely to be those you have heard of or even experienced, including *insomnia* (having trouble falling or staying asleep, which occurs at least occasionally in almost all adults, often during times of stress) and *sleep apnea* (erratic breathing often accompanied by deep snoring, which is common in people with obesity and type 2 diabetes). Some people have issues with staying awake during the day (*narcolepsy*), and others have their sleep interrupted by things like *restless legs syndrome* (when discomfort in your legs as you're falling asleep makes you feel like moving them) or *REM sleep behavior disorder* (which involves acting out your dreams by talking, walking, or swinging your arms).

Insomnia

If you're suffering from insomnia, you're probably experiencing minutes to hours of sleepless time during the night. To deal with it, you may simply need to change your *sleep hygiene* (box 8.3). Also, addressing the thoughts and worries that are keeping you awake in the middle of the night may be in order. Consider "talk therapy" specifically aimed at addressing the issues linked to your insomnia. You may need to learn new ways to manage your negative thought patterns or things you worry about. Many people's short-term insomnia can be treated as effectively with talk therapy as with prescribed meds or sleep aids.

Box 8.3
Improving Your Sleep Hygiene

- Have a routine before bedtime that helps you relax; for example, a hot bath, reading, light yoga, or meditation.
- Try to go to bed and wake up around the same time every day
- Darken the room or use a sleep mask.
- Sleep in a quiet space, and keep it on the cooler side.
- Avoid loud activities or difficult or upsetting conversations just before bedtime.
- Avoid daytime naps if they make it harder for you to fall asleep at your normal time.
- Exercise earlier in the day or evening instead of close to bedtime.
- Avoid eating before bed, especially fatty or heavy foods.
- Expose yourself to sunlight in the morning to reset your circadian rhythm and sleep cycles.

If you've given all these ideas a try and are still having problems sleeping (for reasons that you can't pinpoint), it may be time to schedule a visit with your doctor to see if you have a treatable cause for your sleep issues.

If you feel you need to take something for insomnia or any other sleep issue, talk with your doctor about the best options for you. Some prescription medications are available that may help you with falling asleep and staying asleep. Many aren't recommended for long-term use but some are, such as Ambien, Edluar, Intermezzo, Lunesta, Rozerem, Sonata, and Zolpimist. All have possible side effects, with some resulting in daytime grogginess and sleepiness and others increasing your risk of having a fall. They can also be habit-forming, meaning that you'll have trouble falling asleep without them after a time.

You may also choose to try some over-the-counter sleep aids, including melatonin supplements. Antihistamines can also be used occasionally to induce sleep but are not healthy for long-term use. It's a good idea to seek a medical opinion before taking any drug, as many cause significant side effects, such as daytime sleepiness, dizziness, confusion, cognitive decline, and difficulty urinating. All of these possible symptoms may worsen as you age.

Sleep Apnea

Another common sleep disorder, *obstructive sleep apnea*, is a potentially serious (and sometimes fatal) condition in which your breathing briefly but repeatedly stops and starts during sleep due to the muscles at the back of your throat relaxing and your airway narrowing or closing as you breathe in. Some of its symptoms include snoring loudly, waking up repeatedly, snorting, choking, or gasping while asleep and feeling tired even after a full night's sleep (due to repeated obstructive episodes that prevent deeper sleep). Central sleep apnea is a rarer form that results when your brain fails to send signals to your breathing muscles while you're asleep. Both types are often associated with being older, and they're more common in men. Having excess weight or obesity increases your risk of the obstructive type, which has been linked to high blood pressure, type 2 diabetes, and congestive heart failure—whether it's the cause or the effect—as interrupted sleep can result in higher morning cortisol levels and elevations in blood glucose and insulin resistance.

Some medical options are available for the treatment of sleep apnea. One of the most common is using a continuous positive airway pressure machine (CPAP) at night, but it may also be possible to wear an oral appliance designed to keep your throat open. For milder cases, simply losing some weight or stopping smoking may be enough to help you overcome it. Sleeping on your side rather than your back may alleviate symptoms as well. If nasal allergies are contributing, you may need to talk with your doctor about the recommended treatment for those.

Diabetes, Aging, and Sleep

Last, we really have to talk about how diabetes and aging affect your sleep. There's no doubt that managing your blood glucose levels is a round-the-clock job that takes effort every day—and night. If you think about it, you're trying to manage your glucose while you spend a third of your life asleep.

Anyone who uses insulin knows that blood glucose fluctuations can disrupt your ability to sleep well. If your glucose goes too low, you have to wake up and treat it (and levels tend to go lower at night than usual before you're aware of them). Maybe you're wearing a CGM with alarms that go off with warnings about going too low or even too high (depending on how you set the alarms). Most CGMs have low-glucose alarms that can't be overridden or shut off—for safety reasons. Incessant alarms interrupt many a night's sleep, especially since CGM glucose values lag behind actual blood glucose. And not all those lows are real, as pressure on your CGM sensor from your body while sleeping can result in erroneous "compression lows" that really don't need treatment. Just waking up at night to check your glucose or look at your monitoring device can disrupt normal sleep patterns.

And then there's the aging factor. Most older adults experience changes in the quality and duration of their sleep, even without having diabetes. We mentioned how levels of the natural hormone melatonin decrease with age, which makes deep REM sleep less attainable. Melatonin is normally released when it gets dark and helps promote sleep by coordinating your circadian rhythm. The main brain center in charge of that internal clock, the *suprachiasmatic nucleus* in the *hypothalamus*, is composed of over 20,000 cells that are aging and functioning less efficiently in directing your days and nights, when you feel tired, and when you're alert.

Then add in aches and pains or other chronic issues like sleep apnea, and consistently good sleep can become an impossibility for many people. Those with multiple health conditions are more likely to get fewer than six hours of sleep (when seven to eight hours a night are recommended), have poor sleep quality, and experience symptoms associated with various sleep disorders. Even the medications you take can disrupt sleep, and so many of the older crowd take five or more daily. Their interactions, along with over-the-counter remedies, can have a negative impact on your sleep. If you've tried everything to improve your sleep quality and length and nothing is working, it may be time to check in with your doctor for a holistic review of your health conditions, medications, and possible sleep solutions.

FINDING WAYS TO MANAGE YOUR STRESS

There's no doubt about it: life can be stressful at times. When it comes to managing your blood glucose levels and your health, though, it's more important than ever to find a way to handle your stress before it takes a toll on your body. Both physical and mental stress can raise levels of the hormone cortisol in your blood. We talked some about cortisol back in step 2 related to levels of inflammation and your immune function. Remember that cortisol levels are higher when you're physically or mentally stressed, and chronic stress may even cause you to gain weight.

A lack of sleep can make you more reactive to and less able to handle the curveballs that life throws your way. Trying to sleep when your mind is hyperfocused on your worries and problems can be downright impossible, and you may end up physically fatigued, raising your cortisol levels and making it harder to manage your blood glucose. All of that causes even more stress. You've got to break the cycle.

So take a deep breath. We're all going to need to learn how to relax, no matter what's going on around us, and practice relaxing often (box 8.4).

Diabetes Distress

We all have bad days, but having "diabetes distress" is actually a thing. One in five individuals living with diabetes experiences severe diabetes distress, which is feeling frustrated, defeated, overwhelmed, or burned out by having diabetes and/or its possible health complications and costs of care.[6] It can be a temporary or more permanent emotional state, but it can also turn into depression (refer back to step 7). There are steps you can take to deal with it, though, and you should definitely look into those if you're feeling this way.

The US Centers for Disease Control and Prevention (CDC) has a list of 10 tips on how to cope with diabetes and deal with diabetes distress on its website.[7] Here they are in their entirety:

1. **Pay attention to your feelings.** Almost everyone feels frustrated or stressed from time to time. Dealing with diabetes

Box 8.4
Ways to Relax and Release Your Stress

- Combat your fight-or-flight responses and slow your heart rate by doing three-seven-eight breathing: take three seconds to breathe in deeply, hold your breath for seven seconds, and release it slowly over eight seconds. Repeat at least three times.
- Sit quietly and visualize the stress flowing out of your body while taking deep breaths, slowly inhaling and exhaling while allowing your mind to calm.
- Picture being in an environment that calms you—your happy place—such as sitting poolside, at the beach, or in the woods.
- Try meditating. Sit quietly, breath slowly and deeply, and focus solely on an image in your mind, an object in the room, or a sound.
- Practice using positive affirmations about anything troubling you. For instance, say things such as "I am managing my diabetes," or "I am getting healthy."
- Try progressive muscle relaxation. Start at your toes, tensing and then relaxing them, and then work your way up your whole body, one part at a time.
- Turn on some soothing music, or listen to anything you find relaxing.
- Do yoga and try some yoga deep breathing.
- Get up and move your body however feels best to you. Go for a brisk walk, stretch, do some light calisthenics, or find any activity that calms you down.

can add to these emotions and lead to a sense of being overwhelmed. Having these feelings for more than a week or two may signal that you need help coping with your diabetes.

2. **Talk with your health care providers about your feelings.** Let your doctor, nurse, diabetes educator, psychologist, or social worker know how you've been feeling. They can help you problem-solve your concerns about diabetes. They may

also suggest that you speak with other health care providers to get help.

3. **Talk to your health care providers about other people's negative reactions to your diabetes.** Your health care providers can help you manage feelings of being judged by others because you have diabetes. It is important not to believe that you must hide your diabetes from other people.

4. **Ask if help is available for the cost of diabetes medicines and supplies.** If you are worried about the cost of your medicines, talk with your pharmacist and other health care providers. They may know about government or other programs that can assist people with costs. You can also check with community health centers to see if they know about programs that help people obtain insulin, diabetes medicines, and supplies (test trips, syringes, etc.).

5. **Talk with your family and friends.** Tell those closest to you how you feel about having diabetes. Be honest about the problems you're having. This usually helps to relieve some of the stress. Sometimes the people around you may add to your anxieties, however. Let them know how and when you need them to help you.

6. **Allow loved ones to help you take care of your diabetes.** Those closest to you can help you in several ways. They can remind you to take your medicines, help monitor your blood sugar levels, join you in being physically active, and prepare healthy meals. They can also learn more about diabetes and accompany you on your medical appointments. Ask your loved ones to help with your diabetes in ways that you find useful.

7. **Talk to other people with diabetes.** Others with diabetes understand some of the things you are going through. Ask

them how they deal with their diabetes and what works for them. They can help you feel less lonely and overwhelmed. Ask your health care providers about diabetes support groups in your community or online.

8. **Do one thing at a time.** When you think about everything you need to do to manage your diabetes, it can be overwhelming. To deal with diabetes distress, make a list of all the tasks you must do to take care of yourself each day. Try to work on each task separately, one at a time.

9. **Pace yourself.** As you work toward your goals, such as increasing physical activity, take it slowly. You don't have to meet your goals immediately. You may aim to walk 10 minutes, three times a day each day of the week, but you can start by walking two times a day or every other day.

10. **Take time to do things you enjoy.** Give yourself a break! Set aside time in your day to do something you really love. It could be calling a friend, playing a game with your children or grandchildren, or working on a fun project. Find out about activities near you that you can do with a friend.

You can find these tips and other information online. Go to the CDC's website at www.cdc.gov/diabetes/managing/diabetes-distress/ten-tips-coping-diabetes-distress.html#.

Exercise and Mental Stress

By now you should have figured out that we're both huge proponents of regular physical activity—that is, daily movement in any form you can manage. We've talked about how activity may improve your memory and help your brain heal itself. In fact, it also lowers stress, anxiety, depression, and sleep disorders, all of which are reversible causes of poor memory.[8]

What's more, exercising helps you release fewer stress hormones like cortisol, which will help you relax, sleep better, gain less fat weight, and strengthen your immune system. It also helps you produce more of the better ones, such as *beta-endorphins*, a group of brain hormones that have a calming effect. Ever heard of "runner's high"? That's due to the release of endorphins. You obviously don't have to run to release them; many people benefit from endorphins through swimming and other water exercise (better for your joints too), yoga, walking, and more. Aim for a daily dose of endorphins to relax you and handle your stress. It's also important to manage your physical health when you're regularly active, so let's run to that topic next.

RECOVERING FROM PHYSICAL ACTIVITY OR INACTIVITY

Physical stressors can affect your bodily health in both good and bad ways. For instance, physical activity actually stresses your muscles, joints, tendons, ligaments, bones, and more, pushing them to repair themselves to become stronger and healthier. Every time you complete a workout of any type, you've actually done some damage at the cellular level that must be fixed before you're physically better off. There's a fine balance between doing enough to reap the benefits and overdoing it and causing excessive damage or injury.

Becoming or remaining inactive, though, isn't a great option since it accelerates a loss of muscle, bone strength, and physical functioning that can be difficult to recoup when you're older. Much of our muscular cellular repair occurs with the help of *satellite cells*, but sadly, aging means we have a lot fewer of those around to help us heal quickly than when we were younger. So if you've noticed a longer recovery time after physical activity now that you're older, you're not imagining things.

The importance of sleep and rest cannot be overemphasized. Maintaining healthy sleep habits and routines is necessary for higher-level functioning, mental health, and a healthy weight. In addition, you need to know how to rest and recuperate properly so you can avoid injuries and walk (or cycle or swim) into the sunset of your long and healthy life.

In the last two steps, we'll talk more about health and longevity, including avoiding premature death from cancer or heart disease. And we'll also cover preventing falls and keeping your bones healthy, which—you guessed it—also includes some physical activity. So let's jump right into these final, important topics.

CHAPTER NINE

Step 9: Keep Other Diseases at Bay

Did you know that having diabetes raises your risk of developing many other conditions when it comes to health, such as certain cancers, cardiovascular diseases, dementia, osteoporosis, muscle loss, gum disease, hearing loss, erectile dysfunction, sleep apnea, and other issues? We talked about some of those already in previous steps. Here we'll focus mostly on the first two in that list, cardiovascular diseases and cancer, along with gum disease because your oral health has more of an effect on your overall health than you probably realize (box 9.1). Prevention and early detection are two key components of conquering these diseases.

One of the keys to aging successfully is preventing health problems *before* they happen. That includes the two that Americans are most likely to die from and die from prematurely: cardiovascular diseases and cancers. Almost no diseases are inevitable with diabetes. What you are born with (i.e., your genes) does have some impact that can't be changed, but these diseases have many other causes. And many are preventable or treatable with early detection (box 9.2). So this step is all about understanding what those diseases are and how

232 • AGING WELL WITH DIABETES

Box 9.1

Step 9: Keep Other Diseases at Bay

- What's old
  - Believing that serious diseases, including heart disease and cancer, are a normal part of aging
- What's new
  - Taking steps to prevent additional diseases from developing alongside diabetes
- What you should be doing
  - Practicing healthful behaviors that help you fend off illnesses such as heart disease and cancer by preventing them altogether, delaying the time at which they may affect you, or discovering them early and seeking appropriate treatment

---

to both lower your risk for them and prevent their onset whenever possible despite any elevated risks related to your diabetes.

PREVENTING AND CONTROLLING DISEASE

Taking preventative measures is not as hard as you might think. If you quit smoking, you can significantly reduce your chances of getting heart disease, lung cancer, and other chronic health issues. If you prevent constipation with good eating habits, you can lower your risk of colon cancer. Wearing sunscreen consistently can lower your risk of skin cancer. Small measures can make a big difference. Most of the healthy lifestyle suggestions made throughout the book, when practiced consistently, can help prevent some common illnesses and diseases.

KEEP OTHER DISEASES AT BAY • 233

Box 9.2
Insight from Dr. Munshi

"Health maintenance and disease prevention" is the mantra for healthy aging. What do I think you should be doing along these lines?

- Instead of taking care of diseases, prevention is best. Do what you can by being proactive in preventing some or all of them.
- Stay up to date on your immunizations. Again, an ounce of prevention is worth a pound of cure, as they say.
- Follow your doctors' advice about screenings to catch problems early.
- Continue your good health habits like eating right, exercising, managing your stress levels, and getting plenty of rest.

You will see a list of prevention measures next. Diabetes was included first since you already have that one, but you should already know what you need to do to manage it (based on earlier steps in this book).

Diabetes

- Manage your blood glucose levels.
- Follow a diet high in fiber and low in processed foods.
- Eat a variety of produce of various colors to obtain phytonutrients and antioxidants.
- Exercise regularly.
- Incorporate strength training to build muscle.
- Be physically active on a regular basis, and gain some muscle mass.
- Lose some weight if necessary through diet and exercise.

Heart Disease and Stroke

- Keep your blood pressure in check.
- Quit smoking.

234 • AGING WELL WITH DIABETES

- Lose some excess fat weight.
- Make healthier food choices.
- Eat more omega-3 fats.
- Exercise regularly.
- Drink no more than one to two alcoholic drinks daily for women and men, respectively, or possibly abstain from alcohol altogether.

High Blood Pressure

- Lose some of your excess weight.
- Limit your intake of salt.
- Get enough potassium and magnesium in your diet.
- Be physically active on a regular basis.

Cancer

- Reduce your intake of animal fats and highly processed meats.
- Eat more dietary fiber.
- Minimize your exposure to the sun's ultraviolet rays and radiation.
- Avoid toxic chemicals, including weed killer and insecticides.
- Screen regularly for early detection.

Chronic Obstructive Pulmonary Disease (COPD)

- Quit smoking.
- Live somewhere with lower levels of air pollution.

Osteoarthritis

- Exercise regularly.
- Include moderate resistance exercises to strengthen muscles around affected joints.

Osteoporosis

- Maintain adequate dietary calcium and vitamin D intake.
- Exercise regularly.
- Drink alcohol only moderately (or abstain).
- Cut back on your intake of animal proteins, salt, colas, and caffeine.

Periodontal (Gum) Disease

- Adopt a daily regimen of tooth and gum care that includes flossing, possibly the use of proxy brushes, and daily (or twice daily) brushing with fluoride toothpaste.
- Get regular dental cleanings (at least every six months) and see a periodontist.
- Manage blood glucose levels.

Constipation

- Drink adequate fluids.
- Increase fiber intake.
- Exercise regularly.
- Use the bathroom following meals, when you're helped by reflexes.

Be Proactive about Prevention

It's really up to you to take responsibility for your own health. But what if you don't know what you're supposed to be doing to maintain your health or even the right questions to ask? Next time you visit your doctor, here are some questions you can ask to find out if you're on the right track to prevent unnecessary and avoidable chronic diseases:

- What is my fasting blood glucose, and is it where you think it should be? What about my latest A1C? Should I be doing anything differently to better manage my diabetes at my age?

- What is my blood pressure reading? Is it normal or should it be lower? If lower, how much, and how can I bring it down?
- What is my total blood cholesterol, and how high are the "good" and the "bad" subfractions (HDL and LDL, respectively)? Did the lab break down my subfractions into various categories? What numbers should I be aiming for?
- What is the level of my thyroid hormones, and are they normal?
- How does my weight at this visit compare to the last time I was here? Should I be worrying about my current weight at my age?
- Was my height measurement any shorter than before? How far back in time can you go to compare my height values (and what were they)?
- Do I need to be screened for anything? What about for thinning bones (osteoporosis) or colon cancer?
- Do I need to take all the medications I'm on now? Or can I consider going off any of them or taking lower dosages?
- Are my vaccinations up to date? The current recommendations are to get the following vaccinations:
  - Flu (influenza) shot—every year
  - Prevnar 20 (to prevent bacterial pneumonia)—one dose
  - Tetanus—once every 10 years
  - Shingrix (to prevent shingles, available after age 50)—two doses
  - COVID-19—annual boosters (but talk to your doctor to find out the latest recommendations, especially if you are immunocompromised)
  - RSV (respiratory syncytial virus), for those over age 60, with health conditions, or pregnant—one dose

KEEP OTHER DISEASES AT BAY • 237

You can also check the Centers for Disease Control and Prevention (CDC) website to see other adult vaccines you may want to consider: https://www.cdc.gov/vaccines/schedules/hcp/imz/adult.html.

Stay on Top of Early Screening and Detection

Getting screened for potentially preventable and usually treatable conditions can enhance your health and increase your longevity. Dr. Colberg's family history of colon polyps provides an illuminating example of what prevention can do. It turns out that everyone on her mother's side who has had a colonoscopy (including her brother, aunt, cousins, and others) has had precancerous polyps that were removed during the procedure. She, too, had one removed when first screened at age 50, even though she has a very healthy lifestyle (many cancers have a strong genetic component). Her mother always avoided medical practices, however, preferring herbal supplements and energy healing to basic preventative screenings and regular health care. At age 75, Dr. Colberg's mother had never been screened for polyps and only found out she had colorectal cancer (that had spread to her nearby lymph nodes) when a tumor completely obstructed her colon. She had surgery and radiation therapy but stopped chemotherapy treatments after the first one. She passed away, after the tumor recurred, a few years later of rectal cancer that would likely have been curable with earlier screening and treatment.

This is just one example demonstrating the great deal of control you can have over your own health. No one needs to die from colorectal cancer nowadays, not with our ability to detect and treat it early. According to recent medical trends, more young adults are developing it, so the age for starting regular screenings was recently dropped from 50 down to 45 and possibly earlier if you have a family history or other potential risk factors. The Task Force recommends several colorectal cancer-screening strategies, including stool tests, flexible sigmoidoscopy, colonoscopy, and CT colonography (virtual colonoscopy).[1] It's recommended that adults aged 45–75 be screened for colorectal cancer. Between 75 and 85, it gets riskier to have invasive colon screenings, so your doctor may recommend alternatives or no screening after that point.

Again, screening and monitoring are important keys to maintaining an optimal quality of life, and that includes more than just your blood glucose levels. If you stay on top of your health, you can let your doctor know if you develop new symptoms that should be addressed before they have a chance to become serious and potentially less treatable.

How often you should be screened for various potential diseases depends on your genetic makeup, family history, personal habits, and lifestyle. Ultimately, it is up to you and your doctor to decide what conditions carry the highest risk for you. If a screening test or new symptoms raise any questions about your health, further testing can determine the best course of action, and regular follow-ups can add years to your life.

This approach emphasizes living well even when dealing with diabetes and other chronic health problems. Having good health is not just the absence of disease; it also should include maintaining your physical and mental function (as long as possible) and getting the support you need if any health problems do arise.

HANDLING CARDIOVASCULAR DISEASES

When you have diabetes, your heart health may end up being your biggest worry (box 9.3). Taken together, all cardiovascular diseases are still the leading cause of death for Americans. It's possible to lower your risk of dying early from them, however.

Box 9.3

How Does Diabetes Affect Heart Disease Risk?

Having diabetes is a major risk factor for heart disease and stroke. Older adults with diabetes have a greatly elevated risk of dying from a cardiac event. Overall, up to 80% of people with diabetes die from complications of cardiovascular disease and up to a decade prematurely. The younger you are when you develop type 2 diabetes in particular, the more likely you are to suffer an event: 14 times more likely to have a heart attack and up to 30 times more likely to have a stroke.

The cause is likely underlying systemic inflammation and oxidative stress, which lead to damage to arterial walls and plaque formation around the body. Keeping your blood glucose levels in more normal ranges can help lower your risk, as can tamping down postmeal blood glucose escalations. Using lifestyle improvements including regular physical activity, healthier food choices, and quitting smoking can greatly reduce your risk, along with taking statin medications to lower levels of oxidized, dense LDL cholesterol and total blood fats.

The four most common types are coronary heart disease (which includes heart attack and chest pain), stroke, high blood pressure, and heart failure. Part of lowering your risk is gathering information about your own unique issues and what you can alter on your own. Being physically inactive is a strong risk factor for heart disease, and you can lower or remove it with regular exercise training. Dietary improvements that lower inflammation and boost your antioxidant capacity (which exercise also does) can improve your outcomes, as discussed back in steps 2 and 4. The judicious use of medications for high blood pressure, cholesterol, and glucose may be advised.

Individually, heart disease and stroke are the most common cardiovascular diseases (CVDs) and are leading causes of death and disability for both men and women, accounting for nearly 40% of deaths. Although largely preventable and more likely to occur when you're 65 or older, recent years have seen more CVD-related deaths in younger adults.

Coronary Heart Disease

Blood that supplies your heart muscle with required nutrients and removes waste products flows through a network of coronary arteries. When these blood vessels become narrowed due to the buildup of plaque (which is filled with fat, cholesterol, calcium, immune cells, and more), the blood supply to your heart can be partially or completely blocked. This is coronary heart disease.

Plaque can become fragile and rupture, causing blood clots to form. If they travel downstream and block a coronary artery, the part of the muscle normally supplied by that vessel can infarct, or die, without oxygen. This describes a *myocardial infarction*, otherwise known as a heart attack. Most clots that cause these events occur in arteries about 50% narrowed and often in people with no idea they have any significant plaque buildup.

Early detection gives your doctors the option of trying to open blocked blood vessels using balloon angioplasty or implanted stents, which are devices that hold the vessels open. Many individuals with diagnosed heart disease are put on cholesterol-lowering meds and advised to improve their dietary and exercise habits. Research studies on exercise have shown that plaque buildup may be at least partly reversible with regular physical activity and other important lifestyle improvements.[2] You can modify some of your other CVD risk factors by quitting smoking, lowering your levels of bad cholesterol and other blood fats (see the following sections for which types to focus on), managing your blood pressure, and keeping your blood glucose at more normal levels.

Lowering LDL Cholesterol

Most of the focus on managing blood cholesterol zeros in on *low-density lipoprotein*, or LDL. It's mostly considered bad cholesterol because the oxidation of LDL may be the biggest contributor to plaque formation in arteries. A high level of LDL cholesterol (160 mg/dL and above) is associated with an increased heart disease risk, but it actually depends on your predominant type of LDL.[3]

Small, dense LDL (sd LDL) is preferentially taken up by arterial walls and rapidly oxidized, but large, fluffy LDL is relatively benign. High levels of large, fluffy LDL are common in centenarians, while sd LDL is often associated with high triglycerides and heart disease. Before being treated for elevated LDL cholesterol levels, you may want to have levels of both types measured. If you mainly have the fluffy type, then treatment is not recommended.

Your doctor may also measure your blood levels of lipoprotein (a) and apolipoprotein B, both of which are markers for "bad bad" cholesterol. You're advised to keep your LDL no higher than 120 mg/dL (or under 100 mg/dL with diabetes), particularly if you have mostly sd LDL and your HDL ("good" cholesterol) levels are less than 70 mg/dL.

Aggressively lowering cholesterol levels when you're over 65 should likely be limited to people who have evidence of heart disease, diabetes, or high levels of sd LDL or lipoprotein (a). The drugs of choice are statins (see step 5), as they can block cytokine damage to artery walls and limit plaque formation.

Raising HDL Cholesterol

The other main subtype of cholesterol is *high-density lipoprotein*, or HDL. This type is considered "good," and most people are advised to get their levels as high as possible, especially if their LDL levels are on the high side. Aerobic exercise training has been shown to raise levels of this subfraction, which in turn lowers the risk for plaque formation in arteries around the body.[2] In adults with type 2 diabetes, a recent study showed that both higher HDL levels and a greater time in range (i.e., optimal blood glucose levels) lower the risk of having unstable plaque in coronary (heart) arteries that could form a clot and cause a heart attack or stroke.[4]

Generally, an optimal HDL level is considered anything over 60 mg/dL. At a minimum, though, yours should be 40 mg/dL. There seems to be a maximal benefit to your HDL levels, though: those higher than 90 mg/dL in men and 75 mg/dL in women have not been shown to confer any additional cardiovascular benefits.[5] In fact, if your HDL levels are extremely high—above 100 mg/dL— you might actually have a higher risk of heart disease rather than a lower one.

Peripheral Artery Disease

Related to heart disease is a condition affecting blood flow to your legs known as *peripheral artery disease* (PAD). You can develop plaque in any artery around your body, and PAD occurs in the arteries feeding your legs. Limiting or blocking your blood flow there can cause pain, changes in the color of your skin, sores or ulcers, and difficulty walking. If your leg circulation is totally blocked for a long time, you can experience gangrene in that limb and ultimately lose your toes, foot, or leg to an amputation done in an attempt to save your life. If your doctors can manage your PAD early, though, they can work on restoring the blood flow and function of your limb.

What can you do to manage PAD? Daily walking or other exercise can help, along with taking certain meds that dilate the blood vessels feeding your legs.[6] You may also benefit from surgery that opens those arteries.

Stroke

Like heart disease and PAD, a stroke can result from a clot or blockage of an artery, this time the carotid arteries that carry blood to your brain. This is an *ischemic stroke,* which accounts for over 80% of all strokes. It's also possible to have a *hemorrhagic stroke,* when one of these vessels has a blowout (through a ruptured aneurysm) or is malformed. In either scenario, this type of stroke causes reduced blood flow to the brain through its feeder vessels. Only the areas of the brain that are blood-deprived are affected. If a stroke doesn't kill you, it can leave you badly debilitated and forever changed for the rest of your time on earth. One that affects the back area of your brain can cause vision loss. Other areas of the brain that can be affected control movement, speech, memory, and problem-solving.

What can you do to prevent a stroke? Manage your blood pressure and blood glucose to limit inflammation that can lead to plaque formation. Also, continue to make improvements to your lifestyle that can lower your stroke risk. In older adults, strokes may result from clots forming from abnormal heart rhythms, such as *atrial fibrillation* (or A-fib). Having either type 1 or type 2 diabetes raises your risk of developing A-fib, although more so for adults with type 2. In such cases your doctor may advise you to take a blood thinner to prevent clots from forming. Antiplatelet meds, such as aspirin and Plavix, and anticoagulants such as Coumadin interfere with clotting and may prevent strokes.

If you have any symptoms of a stroke, get to a hospital as quickly as possible to receive tPA (an effective clot-busting drug for ischemic stroke) for the best potential outcome. You must take it within three hours from the onset of your stroke symptoms for it to effectively undo your clot, and very few people make it to the emergency department in time to get this lifesaving treatment.

244 • AGING WELL WITH DIABETES

TIAs, or *transient ischemic attacks*, are basically mini or "warning" strokes that usually result in textbook stroke symptoms and resolve on their own. However, TIAs are strong indicators of a possible major stroke in the future. If you have a TIA, take steps immediately to prevent an actual, more damaging stroke.

High Blood Pressure

To understand what happens when your blood pressure is high, you first need to learn what your blood pressure is (box 9.4). It's quite common for people to have elevations in the first number (systolic) only as they age, and you may only need to keep it below 160 mm Hg at older ages to lower your stroke risk. As you age, you may have poorer health if your blood pressure is too low, but you still want to keep it reasonably controlled, especially with diabetes due to your greater risk of heart problems.

Almost one in three American adults has high blood pressure, many without symptoms, leaving nearly one-third undiagnosed. The incidence is nearly two-thirds in adults aged 65–74. What can you do to lower your blood pressure—whether you've been diagnosed with hypertension or not? First, have your blood pressure

---

Box 9.4
Understanding Blood Pressure

Your blood pressure is the force of the blood pushing against the arterial walls. It is recorded as two numbers, such as 118 over 72 millimeters of mercury (118/72 mm Hg). The first (systolic) number is the arterial pressure during heartbeats, while the second (diastolic) represents the lower pressure that occurs when your heart is at rest between beats. High blood pressure (hypertension) describes a condition in which your blood travels through your blood vessels at pressures consistently above normal.

checked regularly, especially if hypertension runs in your family. If it's high, treat it. Work on reducing your numbers by exercising regularly, possibly cutting back on salt (and increasing your potassium intake), and taking prescribed meds to keep your systolic values below 160 mm Hg. All of these actions can lower your stroke risk. If you leave it untreated, it can cause serious health issues, such as hardened arteries, heart failure, kidney failure, stroke, or heart attack. On the other hand, effectively treating your hypertension dramatically reduces your risk of dire health consequences. A 12- to 13-point reduction in systolic blood pressure can reduce heart attacks by 21%, strokes by 37%, and all deaths from CVD by 25%.

Heart Failure

This condition usually affects the left side of your heart first. That's the side with the two (out of four) heart chambers through which blood flows when it returns from your body or gets pumped out into your arteries or fed through your lungs. Heart failure can happen when even one of the four chambers can't keep up with pumping out all the blood that flows into it. In such cases your blood flow slows down everywhere, causing fluid buildup in various tissues, such as your lungs (*pulmonary edema*). Left heart failure leads to edema of the lungs, while a loss of pumping power on the right side causes blood to back up in your veins, resulting in swelling in your legs and ankles.

What can you do to manage this condition? Heart failure often follows a heart attack when that muscle has been damaged, and it can also result from heart muscle changes due to chronic hypertension. You can work on controlling your risk factors for heart attacks and high blood pressure to prevent heart failure in the first place. If you have it, your doctor can prescribe various drugs to drain excess fluids from the body (diuretics) and increase your heart's pumping ability. Most lifestyle changes have a minimal impact on this condition once you are diagnosed with it, unfortunately, since you can't regain lost heart function. You can make it easier on yourself by keeping your muscles as fit and capable as possible. Even just taking short or frequent walks or moving more lessens the heart's burden of pumping extra blood.

Warning Signs of Heart Attack or Stroke

The most common heart attack symptom is chest pain or discomfort, but women are somewhat more likely than men to experience other symptoms, including shortness of breath, nausea and vomiting, and back or jaw pain (box 9.5). Sadly, women's symptoms are sometimes not taken as seriously when they seek out medical treatment, and heart attacks can be misdiagnosed as other ailments and missed altogether. People with diabetes are also more likely to suffer

---

Box 9.5
Heart Attack Signs and Symptoms

- **Chest discomfort:** constant and in the center of the chest or intermittent. It may feel like bad indigestion, uncomfortable pressure, squeezing, fullness, or acute and stabbing pain.
- **Discomfort elsewhere:** pain or discomfort radiating down one or both arms, the back, the neck, the jaw, or the stomach (referred pain).
- **Shortness of breath:** unusual or unexpected trouble catching your breath, which may be accompanied by chest discomfort.
- **Other symptoms:** sudden sweating, nausea and vomiting, lightheadedness, or unexplained fatigue.
- **No symptoms:** be aware that some individuals have no symptoms; this can lead to misdiagnosis and improper treatment.

KEEP OTHER DISEASES AT BAY · 247

Box 9.6
Stroke Symptoms

- Sudden numbness or weakness, especially on one side of the body (affecting the legs, arms, face, or elsewhere)
- Sudden confusion
- Sudden trouble with normal speaking (slurred speech) or understanding
- Sudden loss of vision in one or both eyes
- Sudden trouble with walking, a loss of balance, or a lack of physical coordination
- Sudden onset of severe headache and dizziness

---

from *silent ischemia,* a reduced blood flow to the heart muscle with no discernible symptoms.[7]

Think "sudden" when it comes to stroke symptoms (box 9.6). Taking immediate action is critical to have the chance to take the clot-busting drug tPA, which can break up a clot and reduce your chances for long-term disability from an ischemic stroke.

Always take any chest pain, discomfort, or other concerning symptoms seriously and seek medical attention immediately. Don't wait more than five minutes after your symptoms start to call for help, and use emergency medical services (EMS) by dialing 9-1-1 to get the fastest treatment (rather than driving yourself or having someone drive you).

PREVENTING AND SURVIVING CANCER

As a person with diabetes, your other biggest worry may be getting cancer. It's second only to CVD as a cause of death. Certain types are more common, such as lung, prostate, colorectal, and skin, but any type can be potentially fatal.

Anyone who has type 2 diabetes is twice as likely to develop liver or pancreatic cancer, and risks are elevated for colon, bladder, and breast cancer as well.[8] If you do develop breast cancer, having diabetes increases your risk of dying from it. For men, though, there appears to be no direct link between diabetes and prostate cancer.

What Is Cancer and How Do You Get It?

Technically, cancerous cells are your own cells that have gone haywire and started reproducing rapidly. This is usually triggered by damage to their DNA. The longer you live, the more likely this will happen, for various reasons. In younger people, the body's natural killer and other immune cells usually destroy cancer cells, but as you age these immune cells decrease. Getting older also leads to longer exposure to pesticides and other toxins that can mutate your DNA, random gene mutations, changes in hormonal levels, and a reduced ability to make bodily repairs. While we don't always know the exact cause of most cancers, it is the most common cause of death in people aged 60–70 and the second leading cause in those over 80.

You aging cells are simply more likely to malfunction, and if they do become cancerous, they may not act or respond in the usual ways that they do in younger people. Many breast tumors actually grow more slowly when you're older, and they may be more responsive to hormone-based treatments. Some other types of cancer, such as acute myelogenous leukemia, respond less well to treatment as you age.

Slow-growing skin cancer is easily treatable (check your moles regularly), while others, such as pancreatic cancer, often escape early detection and have low five-year survival rates. Cancer cells can remain in one area, but when they spread via your blood or lymph

KEEP OTHER DISEASES AT BAY • 249

systems, it's called *metastatic cancer*. If you have cancer, doctors will check the lymph nodes near the cancer site (e.g., in the armpits for breast problems) to determine the extent of the spread (if any). When detected and treated early, most cancers are survivable.

How Can You Lower Your Chances?

What can you do to protect yourself from cancer? Lung cancer, the leading cause of cancer-related deaths and the most common type in anyone over age 60, can often be prevented by not smoking (or quitting) and avoiding exposure to secondhand smoke. The risk for colon cancer, the second leading diagnosis in the over-60 crowd, can be reduced with a healthier diet and regular exercise, and precancerous polyps can be detected (and removed) through regular preventative screenings. Most of the lifestyle changes discussed in previous steps can help you lower your chances of developing cancer (box 9.7). But as you learned from Dr. Colberg's family story, it's also possible to have a strong genetic propensity to develop certain types, something to be aware of in order to plan your screenings accordingly.

For breast cancer in women, regular mammogram screenings and breast self-exams are the best way to find problems early. You can lower your risk by eating less animal fat, drinking less (or no) alcohol, and exercising. Other risk factors may be impossible to change at this point, such as your family history and being childless (or having children after 35), among other things. For cervical cancer, which is strongly linked to human papillomavirus (HPV, a sexually transmitted infection), vaccines are now being recommended for youth and young adults—but us older women have to keep following up with regular pap smear exams to check for it.

Prostate cancer is also common among older men. Their lifetime risk is about 10%, but it's 40 times more prevalent in men between 50 and 85.[9] It appears to be associated with having higher insulin

Box 9.7
Lifestyle Behaviors to Lower Your Risk of Certain Cancers

Proven benefit
- Skin: using sunblock and limiting excessive sun exposure
- Lung, oral, and esophageal: no smoking of cigarettes or chewing of tobacco
- Skin, lung, and so on: avoiding cancer-causing toxins and using protective clothing
- Colon and breast: engaging in physical activity, eating a healthy diet, and possibly taking antioxidants
- Colon, breast, and uterine: keeping body weight within a normal range

Likely benefit
- Colon, lung, and others: eating plenty of fruits and vegetables
- Colon: limiting intake of red meat and highly processed meats (cured lunch meats, hot dogs, and so on)
- Oral, esophageal, breast, and pancreatic: avoiding excessive alcohol consumption

Possible benefit
- Colon, breast: taking folate supplements
- Lung, colon, and prostate: using selenium supplements
- Prostate: taking vitamin E supplements
- Colon, lung, breast, and prostate: eating a balanced diet with citrus fruit, broccoli, leafy vegetables, and fish

levels (i.e., insulin resistance) and more fat weight, so a healthier lifestyle may again be somewhat preventative.

Prostate gland enlargement is also very common with aging, affecting half of men in their 60s and up to 90% of men in their 70s and 80s.[10] This condition is called *benign prostatic hyperplasia*. Although it can cause urinary and other problems (e.g., Dr. Colberg's father gets up every two hours at night to urinate), by itself this enlargement doesn't appear to lead to cancer. Obesity may raise the risk of prostate enlargement, so regular exercise and healthier eating may help prevent it, but given its high prevalence in older men, it's obviously hard to prevent entirely in everyone.

Early and regular screenings can certainly lower your chances of dying from cancers like breast, colon, cervical, and others. Also, be aware of your family history of cancer and assume your risk is higher because of it. Finally, if you develop any of the most common signs and symptoms of cancer as outlined by the American Cancer Society (box 9.8), discuss appropriate approaches to screening and diagnosis with your doctor.[11] And do keep in mind that many signs and symptoms can result from other health issues besides cancer.

By way of example, Dr. Colberg experienced blood in her urine for five days a few years ago and was checked to make sure she didn't have bladder cancer. Since no evidence of that or any other problem was found, it was assumed to be from a kidney stone or other (noncancerous) issue that resolved on its own. It's always worth the peace of mind, though, to be checked to ensure it's not cancer.

How Are Cancers Treated?

The treatment of various types of cancers still includes surgery, radiation, chemotherapy, hormone therapy, bone marrow transplantation, and biotherapy. After a cancer diagnosis, you can discuss treatment options with a cancer doctor (oncologist) to come up with the best plan of action for you and your specific type. Many treatments involve more than one possible therapy.

A delay of a day or two is not going to affect your prognosis, so feel free to seek a second opinion and search for more information online about the various treatment options for your specific type.

Box 9.8
Common Signs and Symptoms of Cancer (American Cancer Society)

- Fatigue or extreme tiredness that doesn't get better with rest
- Weight loss or gain of 10 pounds or more for no known reason
- Eating problems such as a lack of hunger, trouble swallowing, belly pain, or nausea and vomiting
- Swelling or lumps anywhere on the body
- Thickening or lump in the breast or other part of the body
- Pain, especially new or with no known reason, that doesn't go away or gets worse
- Skin changes such as a lump that bleeds or turns scaly, a new mole or a change in a mole, a sore that does not heal, or a yellowish color to the skin or eyes (jaundice)
- Coughing or hoarseness that does not go away
- Unusual bleeding or bruising for no known reason
- A change in bowel habits, such as constipation or diarrhea, that doesn't go away or a change in the appearance of your stools
- Bladder changes such as pain when passing urine, blood in the urine, or needing to pass urine more or less often
- Fever or night sweats
- Headaches
- Vision or hearing problems
- Mouth changes such as sores, bleeding, pain, or numbness

New therapies are being released all the time, but what is best for you may depend on what's available, the stage of your cancer, and your unique health status.

How Can You Improve Your Chances of Surviving Cancer?
Most cancer treatments come with significant side effects, the least of which may be losing your hair (from chemotherapy). You may

also experience chronic fatigue—up to a year after treatment is not uncommon—and lose some of your ability to function normally. You'll need time to recover and recuperate afterward. Certain drugs can help restore your normal immune cells, but the best way to combat side effects is to maintain an active lifestyle—both during and after treatment. You really don't want to lose all the fitness you've worked so hard for, and recouping it gets more difficult with age. If your treatments cause nausea, vomiting, diarrhea, and loss of appetite, try eating small meals every few hours to keep your strength up.

What Are Your Other Options?

When people are faced with a cancer diagnosis, they often seek alternate therapies or healers to "cure" them. While alternative medicine can help some health issues, cancer is not one of them. No supplements have been found that can cure cancer of any type, and some alternate therapies are actually drugs in disguise—and certainly not rated effective or regulated by the US Food and Drug Administration.

Dr. Munshi frequently gives her patients the following advice about using natural remedies for anything that ails them: "If you want to try herbs or a natural cure, try it in its natural form whether it's garlic or cinnamon or turmeric. Don't take pills or powders that are sold in the market or online." Also, if you decide to follow such a therapy while you're dealing with cancer, let your oncologist know because it may be toxic or interact and interfere with your conventional treatment.

Supportive therapies like exercising to boost your immune function and keeping a positive attitude are highly encouraged, however. Turning to prayer or spirituality or other types of emotional support should be sought out whenever desired. It may also comfort you to designate a friend or family member as a patient advocate to guide you through your treatment options if you feel distress or are unable to make those decisions for yourself.

KEEPING YOUR GUMS AND TEETH HEALTHY

Before we close this chapter, we want to address one other health condition that gets talked about far too little because it's not known for being fatal like heart disease and cancer. It's the health of your gums and your teeth. Without treatment, inflamed gums (*periodontitis*) can destroy the bone that supports your teeth, causing them to loosen or fall out completely. We're assuming you'd prefer to keep your teeth and have a healthy mouth, so let's talk more about gum disease and what you can do to prevent or manage it.

What Is the Issue with Gum Disease?

According to statistics from 2021 posted online by the CDC, people with diabetes are much more vulnerable to developing periodontal disease than the average US adult (58% of those with diabetes vs. 38% without).[12] The relationship between the two appears to be bi-directional, meaning that either one can (and does) lead to the other health problem.[13]

A recent study showed that people with type 2 diabetes who frequently brush their teeth have better blood glucose levels—overall (A1C levels), fasting, and after meals—than those who brush less frequently.[14] That means that taking care of your gums and teeth is actually an important part of diabetes self-care. But that level of care doesn't appear to be happening: the CDC also reported that those with diabetes were less likely to use proxy brushes (in spaces between their teeth) or visit a dentist for a cleaning or other preventive care in the past year.[12]

How to Diagnose Gum Problems

Prior studies have confirmed an association between heart issues and gum disease, which doesn't always mean cause and effect but is even more reason to care for your gums on a daily basis. Remember that body-wide, low-level inflammation we discussed back in step 2? Research suggests that periodontal disease may contribute to the progression of other diseases through that very mechanism. In addition to heart disease, diseased gums have been associated with the onset of type 2 diabetes and poor blood glucose management, pneumonia (and other respiratory problems), Alzheimer's disease, rheumatoid arthritis, and even certain cancers. In fact, men with gum disease were found to be more likely to develop kidney cancer (49% more likely), pancreatic cancer (54%), and blood cancers (30%). Talk about fending off the worst health problems if you simply keep your gums in better health (box 9.9)!

Box 9.9
How to Diagnose Gum Problems—Some Symptoms

- Swollen or puffy gums
- Discolored gums (bright red, dark red, or dark purple)
- Gums that are tender to the touch
- Gums that bleed easily (or turn your toothbrush pink after brushing)
- Bleeding caused by brushing or flossing
- Pain when chewing
- Receding gums (making you "long in the tooth")
- Bad breath (*halitosis*) that persists
- Pus between gums and teeth
- New spaces between teeth (triangular, indicating bone loss)
- Changes in your bite (how your teeth fit together)
- Tooth loss or loose teeth

How Can You Improve the Health of Your Gums?

Even if you can't avoid all gum issues, you can certainly stave off some of them and manage any existing problems you do have. It's pretty simple, actually. Follow these easy steps:

- Brush your teeth twice daily with fluoride toothpaste—once in the morning, once in the evening.
- Don't be stingy with your toothbrushes. Replace yours with a new soft one at least every three to four months.
- Floss between your teeth or use an interdental cleaner at least once a day.
- When you have larger spaces between your teeth, clean those using a proxy brush.
- Rinse with an antiseptic mouthwash at least once a day.
- Have regular checkups and dental cleanings.
- If you notice any symptoms of periodontitis, visit a dentist as soon as possible. Time is of the essence to get your gum health under control and reverse damage or prevent more.
- Avoid or limit your intake of sugary snacks and drinks, especially when you won't have a chance to brush your teeth for a while.
- Eat a balanced diet, especially one high in fiber.
- If you smoke, do whatever you can to quit as smoking is associated with having more plaque and tartar and advanced gum disease. (Smoking is also bad for your cardiovascular risk and increases your chances of cancer.)

Even though diabetes raises your chances of cardiovascular disease or certain cancers or other health problems, you can do a great deal to prevent all of them by improving your lifestyle and better managing your diabetes. This step has focused on measures such as

detecting what you can early and taking action and seeking appropriate and timely treatments for your current health concerns. Truly,
your health remains mostly in your own hands. It's your choice to do
what you can to stay as healthy and as happy as you can for the rest of
your (hopefully many) years.

CHAPTER TEN

Step 10: Stay Strong, Stable, and Safe

Now comes the last step, and it's not last because it's the least important. In fact, this step is vital and critical to living well for the rest of your natural life. You probably already know that living into your much older years raises your risk of falling and suffering a serious injury or even death, especially if your bones have thinned a lot. Simply breaking a bone can lead you down the path of long-term health problems and disability. What you may not know is that having diabetes increases your fall risk by up to 17 times.[1] Sometimes the reason for falling is as simple as tripping over dirty laundry on the floor, but for people with diabetes, falls can be related to blood glucose lows or other medication effects. Here we focus specifically on preventing falls and frailty so you can enjoy an independent life well into your later years (box 10.1).

If you become frail, it may be the start of losing your ability to live on your own.[2] The good news is that frailty is largely preventable. Falls are an important potential indicator of frailty. Preventing falls in any and every way possible therefore becomes critical. Falls—particularly those that injure you—often speed up your loss of health and independence. Frailty can be a driver of less physical activity, depression, social isolation, limited functionality, and a diminished quality of life (box 10.2). This is not the path to aging well.

STAY STRONG, STABLE, AND SAFE • 259

Box 10.1

Step 10: Stay Strong, Stable, and Safe

- What's old
  - Expecting to get old and frail and getting badly injured in a fall
- What's new
  - Aging well into your 80s, 90s, and even 100s by preventing falls and frailty and keeping your bones and joints as healthy as possible
- What you should be doing
  - Focusing on the steps you can take to prevent falls, avoid becoming frail, keep your bones stronger, and minimize your joint issues

---

Box 10.2

Insight from Dr. Munshi

When I see people in their 90s who are aging well and living their lives (and they are usually not frail), I don't tell them what to do. Instead, I ask them the secret of their success. Here are some of my patients' most common thoughts:

- Think positively
- Have a reason to get out of bed, whether going to the library, volunteering, caring for a pet, or even going for a walk
- Exercise regularly
- Keep social contact
- Laugh plenty
- Visit with family and friends

LET'S TALK ABOUT FALLS

The statistics of falls are grim. The US Centers for Disease Control and Prevention reports that more than one in four people aged

260 • AGING WELL WITH DIABETES

65 years or older fall each year, and falling is a well-known factor in hip fractures.[3] A fall leading to a hip fracture is a major cause of emergency-department visits for injuries and subsequent hospital admissions, and people with diabetes have an excessive risk of sustaining hip fractures.[4] Even if you aren't injured, falling can lead you to lessen your activity for fear of falling again and limit your mobility over time. Even if you're not experiencing any of these problems yet, you're never too young (or old) to learn ways to avoid them altogether as you inevitably continue to age.

Where Do People Fall Most?

Almost everyone falls down occasionally. Being active actually increases your risk of falling because you're up on your feet doing things. Even if you're physically fit and still have good balance, you may fall for other reasons. Most falls actually occur indoors in your residence, mainly in the bathroom, bedroom, and kitchen (the rooms you use the most). About 1 in 10 falls occur going up and down stairwells, particularly as you walk down. You're more likely to fall on the first and last steps. Since you're more likely to fall at home, your strategy needs to focus on minimizing the impact of a fall when you have one and limiting how often it happens.

Why Do Most People Fall?

Both physical and environmental factors can lead to falls (box 10.3). You're certainly going to have a greater risk of falling if your muscles get weak, especially your thigh muscles. If you have to hurry out of bed and rush to the bathroom in the middle of the night, it's easy to trip and fall. Getting up frequently at night to urinate, even if you're not rushing, can also lead to an accident since the lighting may be dim. People with diabetes often must urinate at night even more frequently when their blood glucose is elevated. Older adults can have

Box 10.3
Causes of Falls in Older Adults

- Poor vision (such as cataracts) and eyewear (including new bifocals)
- Hearing loss
- Incontinence (which may cause rushing to the bathroom)
- Muscle loss (*sarcopenia*) and weakening
- Poor balance and altered gait
- Foot conditions (pain or loss of feeling) and unsafe footwear
- Postural hypotension (blood pressure drop going from sitting to standing)
- Mild cognitive impairment or dementia
- Vascular diseases
- Medications (can cause dizziness or confusion) and polypharmacy
- Declining reflexes
- Thyroid issues
- Safety hazards in the home (such as clutter or uneven floor surfaces) or community

all sorts of visual issues, to boot, including poorer eyesight in dark conditions, floaters, cataracts, diabetes-related eye issues, and more. Even wearing a new pair of glasses—especially if they're bifocals— can throw your balance out of whack. So your goal is to minimize not only the possible causes of falls but also their potential impact by keeping yourself strong and physically active.

What Can You Do to Prevent Falls?

Start with staying active to prevent falls (box 10.4). It may sound counterintuitive to be more active when physical movement can lead to falls, but it's true. You can lower your fall risk with strengthening exercises, particularly for your thigh muscles, and with practicing standing on your tiptoes to build calf and ankle strength. Also work

Box 10.4
Tips to Lessen Your Chances of Falling and Injuring Yourself

- Stay physically active and do muscle-strengthening and balance exercises
- Remove trip hazards from your home (like area rugs)
- Get your vision and hearing tested and corrected where possible
- Read medication labels to be aware of those that cause dizziness
- Get enough rest and sleep to avoid fatigue
- Avoid alcohol
- Stand up slowly to avoid blood pressure drops
- Use a cane or walker to keep you more stable
- Be careful when walking on wet, icy, or uneven surfaces
- Wear supportive footwear (and make it nonskid)

on your flexibility, particularly in your ankles and feet. Exercises like those found in yoga or Pilates can help to strengthen your joints and core muscles while also training your balancing abilities. What's more, your balance ability declines with age and can be made worse by health issues like inner-ear problems and the use of certain meds that can cause dizziness. If you need a refresher on all the balance exercises you can and should be doing regularly, turn back to step 3.

Next, focus on the rest of your physical health. Keeping your feet in better shape can help prevent falls because bunions, calluses, and deformed toes can cause your walking to change or limit your movement. Try to manage your diabetes effectively (so you don't fall from having a low or from needing to urinate more frequently at night with high blood glucose), and be on the alert whenever you develop a new health condition. Talk to your doctor about treating any dizziness you're experiencing, regardless of the cause. Anemia can make you feel weaker, and some cardiovascular problems can make you lightheaded or pass out. If you develop a heart arrhythmia like A-fib (*atrial fibrillation,* which is an abnormal heartbeat very common in older adults) can lead to falls. Even dementia, including Alzheimer's disease, raises your risk of falling (by double) because it can lead you to take shorter steps, sway more, and vary your gait. Many people fall because their walking gait becomes uneven, especially if they have lost some of the feeling in their feet.[5] Be sure to invest in a good pair of shoes that fit comfortably and have stable soles. Simply walking while focusing on something else (which we all do sometimes) can lead to falls, so pay more attention to where you're going. It may be that you simply need to get better glasses to help you see your surroundings.

Also, improve your environment. That means preventing falls by using proper lighting (particularly at night) and removing floor clutter and area rugs. Don't just throw your clothes on the floor when you get into bed as you can trip on them when you get up. Avoid going outside at night where you can't see well unless you take additional lighting with you. You can ask your doctor to have an occupational therapist do a safety assessment of your home to look other potential hazards you can easily remedy.

Finally, if you're prone to falling, don't shy away from using a cane or walker. Many people feel they don't need to lean on a cane, but Dr. Munshi tells them to keep it with them anyway. If you ever feel imbalanced, lean on it or gradually sit down on the floor—instead of possibly falling and breaking something. Also remember that it's better for you to use a cane or walker if that's the only way you'll keep active (rather than avoid walking because you are afraid of falling.) Having a hip fracture or other broken bone often puts you on a slippery slope of declining health and is best avoided in any way possible.

LET'S TALK ABOUT FRAILTY

What does it mean to be "frail"? Basically, it's when you have such a diminished physical capacity that you can no longer handle the activities of daily life on your own. It usually involves a decline in your mobility, stability, and strength. It can lead to being less socially active, falling more, becoming more prone to bone fractures, experiencing incontinence, having cognitive impairment, and losing much of your quality of life. A working definition of frailty from aging specialists is the following: if you have experienced excessive or rapid weight loss, are exhausted, have a weak grip strength, walk slowly, and have low levels of physical activity, then you're likely frail.

Can Frailty Be Predicted?

Just looking at how well you perform basic activities of daily living once you hit 70 years of age is a decent predictor of frailty. If you can use the bathroom, wash, bathe, dress yourself, feed yourself a meal, and control your bowels, you're not frail. Once you can no longer do these basic activities, your risk of dying within six months is over 50%. If you survive that half year, you're likely to be compelled to live in a nursing home or have extensive help at home. In other words, simply being able to take care of yourself is a much better predictor of frailty than having any particular disease.

What Causes Someone to Become Frail?

Most of your physiological system peaks in your mid-20s and then starts a slow, steady decline over your lifetime. This includes your vision, hearing, sense of smell, appetite, hormone levels, bone minerals, muscle mass, memory, and more. This decline can be sped up by health conditions that are not well managed, and it can be slowed by many of your lifestyle choices. Contributing factors to a faster decline include nutritional deficiencies, visual problems, too many medications, a loss of balance ability, fitness declines, low iron levels (anemia), heart failure, thinning bones, muscle loss (sarcopenia), chronic pain, and extended bedrest.

The quickest way to become frail is through muscular weakness caused by muscle wasting, so ensure you train for good muscle health (refer back to step 3 for tips). One of the best measures of declining abilities is your handgrip strength—and, coincidentally, it's also a good predictor of mortality. So keep those hands strong, and the rest of you as well.

About half of the people who suffer from muscle wasting also have obesity, so in this case a little extra weight won't help you. In fact, excess fat weight when you're losing muscle strength is a recipe for disaster. That combination is a great predictor of becoming frail at a younger age.[6] It's hard enough to move a heavier body around with strong muscles, but when you lose your strength, it can be virtually impossible and severely limit your mobility. In particular, when your excess fat is stored around your middle, the extra release of cytokines (see step 2) adds to your risk of inflammation, insulin resistance, hypertension, elevated cholesterol, and heart disease, all of which are linked to frailty.[7] The best way to prevent all of them is to regularly use your body, eat well, and exercise your brain.

Is Frailty Reversible?

We already know that frailty may be largely preventable, but can you reverse it once you have it? It can be difficult to completely reverse, but you can take steps, including the following, to improve your physical functioning:

- Maintain your food intake to avoid further muscle loss.
- Make your diet a healthy one.

- Increase your fitness and strength by including resistance exercise.
- Work on your balance and flexibility.
- Do more spontaneous physical activity during the day.
- Limit TV watching and sedentary pursuits.
- Keep your mind active doing puzzles, brain games like sudoku, reading, or learning something new.
- Seek help for signs of depression, anxiety, or chronic pain.
- Have your eyes and ears checked regularly and address any issues.
- Go over your medications regularly with your doctor and eliminate anything that might be unnecessary, adjusting levels when appropriate.
- Get checked for anemia (hemoglobin level below 12 mg/dL) if you experience dizziness with standing. Anemia can be reversed with the use of recombinant erythropoietin or darbepoetin to boost your red blood cells.
- Have your hormone levels tested; you may also consider getting testosterone replacement therapy to help restore your muscle mass.

LET'S TALK ABOUT BONE HEALTH

In addition to grip and muscle strength, having healthy bones and joints is critical for remaining mobile and pain-free. Like the other bodily systems in decline, your bones have been losing some of their mineral deposits throughout your adulthood. Having perilously thin bones is called *osteoporosis*, but just as prediabetes occurs before the onset of type 2 diabetes, a lesser demineralization state known as *osteopenia* happens before full-blown bone thinning.

Close to half of all Americans older than 50 are considered to be at risk for fractures from osteoporosis and low bone mass, particularly hip fractures, although spine and wrist fractures are also common. Low bone density at either the hip (femur neck) or lower (lumbar) spine or both was 43.1% among adults aged 50 and over and 47.5% for anyone 65 and over; more women have significant bone loss than men.[8]

Once your bone mass reaches a critical level, bone fractures can occur and recur from seemingly minor impacts. Most women start out with bones that are less dense than men's, so they often feel the effect of this thinning process sooner than men, particularly after menopause. So let's talk about what you can do to prevent these problems or deal with them if you already have thin bones.

Who Is Most Likely to Get Osteoporosis?

Since bone thinning happens slowly over many years, the older you get, the greater your chances for developing osteoporosis.[9] Once you reach a critically low bone mineral density, your chances of having fractures and experiencing some disability rise tremendously. Being female and going through menopause early (the average age is around 51 years old in the United States) increases your odds because the loss of estrogen, the primary female hormone, contributes to faster bone demineralization. After menopause, women lose bone at an average rate of 2%–3% per year, while men the same age lose less than half a percent.[10] Part of the risk is hereditary, and people with a small frame or who are Caucasian or Asian are more likely to develop osteoporosis.[8] Women with diabetes—type 1 in particular—are even more likely to lose bone minerals faster than the norm.[11] Prolonged immobilization also has a profoundly bad impact on bone health. Some of your chances of developing osteoporosis, however, are affected by your lifestyle choices, including

268 • AGING WELL WITH DIABETES

smoking, drinking excessively, eating a poor diet, and living a sedentary life.

How Do You Know If You Have It?

The most visible sign of bone loss is a gradual shortening in overall height with age, which happens due to compression of the vertebrae in your back. Your bone mass peaks somewhere in your mid-20s and then starts to decline in your thigh bones (femurs). Those losses are followed by spinal changes in your next decade of life and the loss of arm-bone minerals in your 40s. Men are about a decade behind women in developing osteoporosis, but if they do fracture a hip, they're twice as likely to die early compared to a woman with a similar fracture. People with excess body fat and muscle mass loss are even more likely to break a hip.[12]

To assess your bone status, you can have painless, noninvasive bone mineral density scans done with methods like single-photon absorptiometry, dual-photon absorptiometry, dual-energy X-ray absorptiometry, computed tomography scanning, and ultrasound. Women should have their bone mineral density measured around menopause to establish a baseline and at least once more at age 65, men, when they reach 65–70. A bone mineral density of more than 2.5 standard deviations below the young adult average (a T-score of 1.0–2.5) is considered osteoporosis. Osteopenia can also be diagnosed with the same scans, along with your annual risk of suffering a fracture in various areas of the body. Repeat testing every two years to follow your rate of bone loss.

Can Osteoporosis Be Prevented or Reversed?

The best prevention for prematurely thin bones is probably having as high of a peak bone mass as you could during your 20s, which could have been accomplished with regular weight-bearing exercise, resistance training, and a healthy diet containing plenty of calcium. If that ship has already sailed with time (like it has for the majority of us), then your best bet is to slow the rate of decline in any way possible. If you're a postmenopausal woman, you may benefit (for a short while) from estrogen-replacement therapies, but those have their drawbacks.

Strategies for treating osteoporosis are similar to those for preventing it. Get adequate amounts of calcium in your diet; get some sun exposure or take vitamin D supplements; positively stress your bones with the right types of physical activity, like low-impact (not no-impact) exercise; and consider using medications that promote bone health.[10,13] If your osteoporosis stems from an underlying health condition (like an overactive parathyroid gland), your doctor can treat that disease to improve your bones.

Studies have examined different types of physical activity and determined that you should be doing regular, moderate weight-bearing exercise, such as walking or aerobics, that strengthens bone and may increase bone formation. Resistance or weight training also promotes healthy bones. Even though the benefits may be few, at least it leads to a gain and not a loss of bone minerals, such as inactivity brings. Even if you can't completely prevent or reverse bone mineral losses, you can slow them down.

How Important Is Calcium?

For decades, the recommendation was to take in more calcium to slow bone thinning. There's no doubt that getting enough calcium when your bones are reaching their peak minerals is crucial. Doctors used to recommend that older women in particular take calcium supplements to boost their overall intake, and during those times, manufacturers starting adding calcium to products like orange juice.

The scientific findings have been changing, however, and it's now less certain whether extra calcium intake after menopause has much

270 • AGING WELL WITH DIABETES

impact on bone loss when taken by itself. Up through age 50, most people should get 1,000 mg daily through dietary sources. Between 50 and 70, women should get 1,200 mg, and then at age 71, men join them at that level of intake.[10]

Vitamin D has taken on greater importance since it increases the absorption of calcium from the gut and helps it infiltrate the bones. You can usually get what you need from 10 to 15 minutes of sunlight without sunscreen a couple of times a week, just on your hands and face. It's difficult, however, to get much of this vitamin through food or sunlight exposure in some cases (with older or darker skin), so it can be taken as a supplement. In foods, vitamin D in found in fatty fish like salmon, tuna, and mackerel; fish liver oils (e.g., cod liver oil); and liver, cheese, and egg yolks. Margarine, milk, and cereals are often fortified with it. The recommended intake is 800 international units a day for anyone over 70. Acting as a hormone, vitamin D has impacts on tissues around the body, the bone being just one of them. Recent research has reported that calcium supplements may lead to a 1% increase in bone density in the first year of use only, and vitamin D supplements only help in people with low blood levels to start with (so they're not recommended for everyone).[14] Supplementing with vitamin D_3 plus calcium daily has been shown to help prevent fractures, along with other lifestyle changes.[15]

There is increasing evidence that too much calcium from supplements is not likely to be beneficial and may actually harm you. Accordingly, most calcium should come from what you eat (table 10.1). Dairy products are high in calcium, but some people avoid dairy due to lactose intolerance or a vegan lifestyle. Many lactose-free products are readily available nowadays for those with lactose issues, and a number of dark-green leafy vegetables contain a good deal of calcium that is well absorbed, including kale, mustard and turnip greens, broccoli, and Brussels sprouts. Legumes (like pinto, navy, and black

Table 10.1. Food Sources and Absorption Rates of Calcium

Food source	Calcium (milligrams)	Absorption (%)
Milk, 1 cup	250–300	32
Most cheeses, 1.5 ounces	305–336	32
Yogurt, low fat, 8-ounce container	338–448	32
Soy milk, calcium fortified, 1 cup	75–300	24
Tofu, 1/2 cup	130 (medium), 258 (firm)	31
Pink salmon, canned, with bone, 3 ounces	181	27
Sardines, Atlantic, in oil, drained, 3 ounces	325	27
Rainbow trout, farmed, cooked, 3 ounces	173	27
Ocean perch, Atlantic, cooked, 3 ounces	116	27
Most canned beans, 1 cup	69–161	17
Turnip greens, boiled, 1 cup	198	52
Bok choy, boiled, 1 cup	158	54
Spinach, boiled, 1 cup	244	5
Kale, boiled, 1 cup	94	59
Mustard greens, boiled, 1 cup	82	58
Broccoli, boiled, 1 cup	178	53
Brussels sprouts, boiled, 1 cup	56	64
Cauliflower, boiled, 1 cup	34	69
Almonds, dry roasted, 1 cup	80	21
Orange juice, calcium fortified, 1 cup	300	25

beans) and foods made from soybeans, like tofu, are also rich in calcium. Plant foods are also rich in phytochemicals and antioxidants while containing little fat, no cholesterol, and no animal proteins that may actually cause bones to lose calcium. Consider both the calcium content of various foods as well as how much of it is bioavailable when making food choices.

It is possible to take in too much calcium, but that rarely happens from dietary sources. Excess intake is typically related to using supplements and excess antacids. If you get more than 4,000 mg per day, you can end up with calcium toxicity, which can damage your kidneys and cause calcium deposition, along with increasing your risk of kidney stones and constipation.

What Else Affects Your Bone Health?

Phosphorus: Other food and beverage choices can also have an impact on your bones. For example, your intake of the mineral phosphorus (also stored in bones as part of calcium-phosphate salts) should be balanced with an equal intake of calcium, but many people take in huge amounts of phosphorus through dark-colored colas and other consumables. Colas have high amounts of phosphoric acid and, in excess, that can lead to bone mineral losses, as can the caffeine in most sodas. Being unbalanced in your intake of both can trigger parathyroid hormone release, which can lead to calcium being leached from bones.[16]

Protein: While once the opposite was believed, the current consensus is that protein intake is good for bone health. A protein-rich diet, provided you're getting adequate amounts of calcium, benefits the health of bones, even in older adults who have osteoporosis. It doesn't seem to matter whether the protein comes from plants or animal sources either.

Salt: A high amount of salt in your diet is another story. It helps control the amount of calcium in the bones, and it's thought that consuming too much salt can lead to bone weakening and osteoporosis. So "protein good, salt bad" in this context.

Are Any Medical Treatments Available?

Supplemental estrogen may benefit women's bone health, but it had been recommended for only up to five years after menopause and not after age 60 due to potential negative side effects. Recent research reverses this somewhat and indicates that low-dose and transdermal hormone therapy (with estrogen) is safer than the oral doses and may be appropriate for some women to treat osteoporosis.[17] Males with low testosterone levels may need to take testosterone to protect their bones.

Medications used to treat excessively thin bones include bisphosphonates, which slow the breakdown of bone. The most common include the following:

- Fosamax (weekly pill)
- Actonel (weekly or monthly pill)
- Boniva (monthly pill or quarterly intravenous [IV] infusion)
- Reclast (annual IV infusion)

Many of these meds are also offered as cheaper generics—ask your doctor about those alternatives as well. Keep in mind that due to the potential side effects of long-term use of these medications, you may need a break from them after five years. The positive effects seem to last even during breaks, though, as the meds build up in your bones.

Some medications in a different class are recommended to anyone who can't take a bisphosphonate, such as those with reduced kidney function:

- Prolia or Xgeva (injection under skin every six months)

Even more medication choices, including the following, actually build bone rather than slow its breakdown:

- Forteo (daily injection)
- Tymlos (daily injection)
- Evenity (monthly injection for one year)

These types of drugs are usually only used when you have very low bone density, have had fractures, or have steroid-induced bone loss. You shouldn't take them if you have a high risk of bone cancer, and all are taken for only one to two years before you should cycle onto one of the bisphosphonates to keep your bones stable.

LET'S TALK ABOUT JOINT HEALTH (ARTHRITIS, IN PARTICULAR)

Let's face it—it's hard to be mobile if your joints aren't working well for you. More than 15 million Americans have some chronic joint problems, possibly related to osteoarthritis (the most common type of arthritis), rheumatoid arthritis, psoriatic arthritis, or another of the 100 forms of arthritis and related diseases.[18] The most common is *osteoarthritis*, the painful inflammation of a joint or joints in your body caused by degeneration of the bony surfaces and most often occurring in your knees, hips, spine, fingers, and toes. It's possible to develop other joint issues as well that can have a dire effect on your quality of life. In this section, we'll mainly focus on osteoarthritis for simplicity's sake.

How Do Joints Work with and without Arthritis?

You have to have joints to move. *Tendons* that form the ends of muscles cross joints to allow you to contract and move those areas, and *ligaments* cross joints from bone to bone to keep them stable and in place. The bones involved in joints are covered with cartilage on the ends where they meet and interact, and this covering acts as a cushion that allows joints to move smoothly and painlessly.

When you cause undue damage to the joint, however, the cartilage surfaces become swollen (inflamed) and painful, forming tiny crevasses that hinder movement. As the cartilage loses some of its elasticity, it's likely to sustain more damage and may form bone spurs. The synovial fluid in the middle of joints, tendons, and ligaments, can also become inflamed. If and when you lose all the cartilage surface, your joint's mobility will be severely limited, and you'll experience near-constant pain and discomfort when you move.

Who's going to get arthritis? If you're carrying around extra fat weight, your lower extremity joints are more likely to suffer due to the extra stress you're putting on the cartilage in your hips and knees. More than half of all adults with diabetes have some osteoarthritis.[19] If you've injured one of your joints in the past—for instance, playing contact sports—it's more likely to develop arthritis as you age.

What Are the Symptoms of Arthritis and Other Joint Issues?

The symptoms of osteoarthritis are easily identifiable and undeniable (box 10.5), although their severity can differ depending on which joint is affected and vary from person to person. Your pain and symptoms may worsen after you use your joints all day or after long periods of little movement.

With knee arthritis, it's possible that your joint may lock up when you step up or down or bend it. If it's in your hip, you could have osteoarthritis or rheumatoid, psoriatic, or post-traumatic arthritis, although the most common cause is wear and tear to your hip joint over time. It's possible that you may feel pain in or around your hip, stiffness, clicking noises when moving, and muscular weakness. As with knees, your hips can lock up on you during movement. In people with diabetes, limited joint mobility in hips and shoulders (that is, "frozen" joints) can result from long-term damage related to elevated blood glucose levels.

Box 10.5
Osteoarthritis Signs and Symptoms

- Joint pain, made worse by cool, damp weather
- Crackling or popping in arthritic joints
- Enlarged, swollen joints that often feel tender when touched
- Stiffness and restricted movement in affected joints
- Unstable joints that move too far or in the wrong direction

If you develop arthritis in your finger joints, you may have reduced strength and movement in your fingers and hands, making tasks like buttoning clothes or opening the lids of jars difficult. Arthritic finger joints can have hard, bony enlargements, but you can also have pain and movement limitations in your fingers and hands related to other common conditions experienced by anyone with long-standing diabetes, including trigger finger and Dupuytren's contracture.[20]

If your spine is affected by arthritis, you may have neck and low back pain, along with weakness and numbness. Over time, it's also possible to have compression of the spinal vertebrae related to thinning bones (see earlier in this step), which can result in spinal pain as well.

Why Do Arthritic Joints Hurt?

The pain from osteoarthritis emanates from irritated nerves in adjacent stretched or inflamed areas—since cartilage itself contains no nerves. Your pain may be "referred," meaning that you feel it somewhere other than directly in the joints with arthritis. If you develop advanced arthritis, you may have continuous pain. This happens when you've lost almost all or all of the cartilage cushion in affected joints.

Some people have told us that they can sense changes in the weather based on the pain and stiffness in their arthritic joints. They claim that, in general, their muscles, ligaments, and joints are stiffer and more painful with damp and cold conditions and better with warmer, drier weather. While studies have had a hard time proving this association (since so many other factors can affect how much pain we are feeling), it's still good advice to relieve joint pain by staying active no matter the weather.

Does Exercising Hurt Arthritic Joints?

While you can certainly irritate your joints doing intense activities that cause injury to your joint surfaces, most easy to moderate-intensity activities will help rather than hurt joints.[21] Include specific training exercises that strengthen all the surrounding muscles that support and protect any of your affected joints. For instance, for knee issues strengthen both groups of muscles that cross that joint (the quadriceps muscles in the front of your thighs and the hamstrings in the back).

You can also try relieving pain and stiffness with warm-water therapy (more reason to get a hot tub), regular stretching, yoga, and easy or moderate walking. You may also enjoy some activities that don't require you to put weight on painful joints, such as cycling, water sports, and seated resistance training. Remember to always stretch affected joints as well to keep them as mobile as possible.

How Are Painful Joints Treated or Managed?

As we just discussed with regard to staying active, most treatments for affected joints focus more on practical ways to manage pain without medication. In addition to exercising moderately, you can try any of the following:

- Massage therapy (of surrounding muscles)
- Heat packs or cold packs (when painful or after exercise)
- Athletic tape or supports (for arthritic knees in particular)
- Orthotics or wedged shoe insoles (especially with leg-length discrepancies)
- Weight loss (with exercise included)
- A walking stick, cane, or other support

If you think you need medications to manage the pain, there are several types you can try, with various benefits and downsides to each:

Nonprescription pain relievers: You can certainly try the judicious use of nonprescription pain relievers such as acetaminophen (Tylenol), but watch out for liver damage caused by taking too much of it (plus, it's not anti-inflammatory). People also frequently use NSAIDs (otherwise known as *nonsteroidal anti-inflammatory drugs*), such as ibuprofen (sold as generics, Advil, or Nuprin), naproxen (Aleve), and aspirin in recommended doses. Just be aware of the potential for stomach irritation from NSAID use in particular, along with blood thinning. They can also damage your kidneys and thin your blood when you use them long term, and you would probably need to since arthritic pain usually sticks around. It can benefit you to take some of these pain meds prophylactically, as a preventative or protective measure, to prevent joint irritation and swelling. Taking the pain control med before the pain starts can also improve your ability to be active. If you need these medications frequently, it would be prudent to check with your doctor about how their use may affect any other health issues you have or could develop.

Prescription pain medications: If your pain is extreme, you may need stronger prescription pain meds, but use these with caution because some of them may be addictive (opioids in particular) or cause other health problems. Celecoxib (Celebrex) is a prescription NSAID used to treat mild to moderate pain and help relieve the symptoms of various types of arthritis, including inflammation, swelling, stiffness, and joint pain. Although it may have beneficial effects beyond pain (lowering blood glucose and lessening memory defects), it can also raise potassium levels too high and damage your kidneys.

Corticosteroids: Sometimes called steroids or glucocorticoids, these reduce inflammation by acting like your natural hormone cortisol. They work quickly and provide short-term relief (in pill or injection forms), but long-term use can cause weight gain, cataracts, high blood pressure, osteoporosis, and sky-high blood glucose levels. If you need to take them for a long time for pain management, you should only be prescribed a small amount each day. Many other meds are prescribed for rheumatoid arthritis. Also, because pain meds have the potential to interact with other drugs, talk with your doctor about any new symptoms you develop and whether they could be related to your pain management meds.

Can Food or Supplements Heal Joints?

Some dietary changes may help joint pain somewhat. Research has shown that omega-3 fats (through fish and certain nuts) and plant-based antioxidants may lower inflammation. Claims about other anti-inflammatory and antioxidant spices like ginger, holy basil, green tea, rosemary, scutellaria, huz hang, and turmeric have certainly been made, but none have been unequivocally proven to be effective. Turmeric's most active component, curcumin, is a proven powerful anti-inflammatory and antioxidant, but unfortunately, most turmeric spice only contains 2%–6% curcumin. Research has shown some anti-pain benefits to taking high-quality extracts of curcumin, but more studies are needed.[22]

Others have tried herbal remedies for arthritis, such as glucosamine and chondroitin. Glucosamine is supposed to repair wear and tear to cartilage surfaces, but most well-conducted studies have shown limited or no effects on arthritic joints. Likewise, chondroitin is purported to protect cartilage and increase its ability to absorb shock, but study results have been equivocal.[23]

Plus, there are potential downsides to using unregulated herbal supplements. Studies in lab animals at one point reported that glucosamine can destroy insulin-producing pancreatic cells and is linked to the development of diabetes—although it's not clear whether this happens in humans. Chondroitin may interact with blood thinners, such as warfarin, and increase your risk of bleeding. The US Food and Drug Administration does not regulate supplements at all (unless people start dying from using them), and you never know what you're getting when you buy them. They may or may not contain the amounts stated on the label, or they could be contaminated—and they are never covered by health insurance so you'll have to pay for them yourself.

Do Arthritic Joints Need Surgery?

At this point you probably know, or have heard about, quite a few older adults who have undergone arthroscopic surgery to repair their joints or have total joint replacements. Not everyone's joints worsen over time, and they often deteriorate very slowly, giving you time to weigh your options. When you reach a point where your joint pain is severe and nearly chronic and limits your mobility, surgery may be best. More and more people are finding that knee and hip replacements are quite effective at alleviating the majority of their joint issues. Many types of surgical procedures are available to treat different joints, the most well-known being artificial joint replacement for completely damaged cartilage surfaces. You may be able to undergo less dramatic surgical intervention to treat osteoarthritis in its early stages and slow its progression. Surgical techniques are becoming more reliable every day due to new bone substitutes, specialized alloys, and innovative designs for replacement joints. In the near future, you may be able to look forward to minimally invasive joint-replacement surgeries.

We've covered a lot of ground in this last important step on your journey to a healthier, long life with diabetes in your later years. You've learned the importance of preventing and managing falls, preventing frailty, keeping your bones stronger and less likely to fracture, and working with your aging joints. As your mobility is so important to living well and independently, it's not a step to be taken lightly. All we must do now is wrap up all we've discussed, which we'll do next.

Final Thoughts

Congratulations! You've made it through all 10 steps to help you age well with diabetes, and you now possess the knowledge to live the rest of your wonderful life to the fullest and with the best possible health. While we know you still have to put all these steps into practice, we think you've got this! Changing lifelong habits can be a bit challenging, but you can always refer back to this book and take it step by step—it's a marathon to the finish, not a sprint. Even if you make just very small changes over time, you'll see the effects start to accumulate in your enhanced health and quality of life. Here we've summarized for you in one list the main points covered in this book to set you on the path to a new way of thinking:

Step 1: Change Your Sweetness
- Work with your health care team to personalize your blood glucose targets depending on your overall health, chance for lows, and more.
- Don't be afraid to let some of the numbers rise when you are trying to avoid lows. All high numbers are not the enemy. It's the persistent highs that you should guard against.

Step 2: Reverse Your Road to Diabetes
- Focus on the lifestyle habits that will actually increase the length of time you can live well, along with those that improve your blood glucose and level of insulin resistance, lower your blood pressure, and benefit your cholesterol levels to achieve better heart health.
- Lower your risk of chronic inflammation to fend off future health complications.

Step 3: Stand Up and Stride Away

- Work on becoming and staying as physically active as you can in any and every way possible.
- Include various types of physical activity every week to enhance your longevity and quality of life.
- Exercise smarter and allow yourself enough time to recover to avoid injuries.

Step 4: Boost Your Gut Health and Your Diet

- Make food choices (and other lifestyle changes) that contribute to the health and integrity of your gut, which will benefit your overall health and your blood glucose levels.
- Prevent and correct nutritional deficiencies to boost bone and heart health.

Step 5: Take a Medication Inventory

- Talk with your health care team about ways to simplify your medication regimen, especially if you take four or more pre-scribed meds daily.
- Always provide your current list of meds to your doctors, and include any over-the-counter medications, herbs, and supplements.

Step 6: Achieve Your Desired Body Weight

- Talk with your health care team about safely losing fat from the right places and maintaining your new weight.
- Learn how to build up muscle strength and resist muscle loss while dieting to improve your stamina and mobility.

Step 7: Rev Up Your Brain Power

- Take action to improve your brain power and memory to retain your independence.
- Discover ways to stay mentally healthy and combat depression

Step 8: Sleep Well, Rest, and Recuperate

- Improve your sleep hygiene for quality sleep to ensure better health with diabetes and other chronic conditions.
- Find ways to rest, including power naps, restful activities, and mental rest and relaxation.

Step 9: Keep Other Diseases at Bay

- Practice healthful behaviors that help you fend off illnesses like heart disease and cancer by preventing them altogether or finding them early and seeking appropriate treatment.
- Improve the health of your gums to promote overall wellness.

Step 10: Stay Strong, Stable, and Safe

- Focus on the steps you can take to prevent falls, avoid becoming frail, keep your bones stronger, and keep you living independently for longer.
- Understand arthritis and joint issues and how to prevent and treat them.

In the end—and the reason you likely read this book—you're trying to maintain your functionality and independence for as long as possible, along with enjoying a higher quality of living for as long as you live. You probably want to increase your life span and savor every bit of life you have left. That should be less of a problem now that you have all the latest information possible on how to do it—even with diabetes as your constant companion. So question your doctor's opinion, continue to educate yourself, be your own advocate, seek happiness, enjoy life, and smile (with healthy teeth and gums) all the way to the century mark and beyond!

Notes

CHAPTER 1

1. Centers for Disease Control and Prevention. National diabetes statistics report. 2023. Accessed August 1, 2024. https://www.cdc.gov/diabetes/php/data-research/index.html
2. American Diabetes Association Professional Practice Committee. Diagnosis and classification of diabetes: standards of care in diabetes—2024, part 2. *Diabetes Care.* 2024;47(suppl 1):S20–S42. https://doi.org/10.2337/dc24-S002
3. American Diabetes Association Professional Practice Committee. Older adults: standards of care in diabetes—2024, part 13. *Diabetes Care.* 2024;47(suppl 1):S244–S257. https://doi.org/10.2337/dc24-S013
4. Watkins DA, Ali MK. Measuring the global burden of diabetes: implications for health policy, practice, and research. *Lancet.* 2023;402(10397):163–165. https://doi.org/10.1016/s0140-6736(23)01287-4
5. American Diabetes Association Professional Practice Committee. Glycemic goals and hypoglycemia: standards of care in diabetes—2024, part 6. *Diabetes Care.* 2024;47(suppl 1):S111–S125. https://doi.org/10.2337/dc24-S006
6. American Diabetes Association Professional Practice Committee. Diabetes technology: standards of care in diabetes—2024, part 7. *Diabetes Care.* 2024;47(suppl 1):S126–S144. https://doi.org/10.2337/dc24-S007
7. Cowart K, Updike WH, Franks R. Continuous glucose monitoring in persons with type 2 diabetes not using insulin. *Expert Rev Med Devices.* 2021;18(11):1049–1055. https://doi.org/10.1080/17434440.2021.1992274
8. Grammes J, Schmid S, Bozkurt L, et al. Continuous glucose monitoring in older adults with diabetes: data from the diabetes prospective follow-up (DPV) registry. *Diabet Med.* November 27, 2023;41(3):e15261. https://doi.org/10.1111/dme.15261
9. Leite SAO, Silva MP, Lavalle ACR, et al. Use of continuous glucose monitoring in insulin-treated older adults with type 2 diabetes. *Diabetol Metab Syndr.* November 23, 2023;15(1):240. https://doi.org/10.1186/s13098-023-01225-4

CHAPTER 2

1. Cantley NW, Lonnen K, Kyrou I, Tehrani AA, Kahal H. The association between overweight/obesity and double diabetes in adults with type 1 diabetes: a cross-sectional study. *BMC Endocr Disord.* 2021;21(1):187. https://doi.org/10.1186/s12902-021-00851-1

2. Ho TP, Zhao X, Courville AB, et al. Effects of a 12-month moderate weight loss intervention on insulin sensitivity and inflammation status in nondiabetic overweight and obese subjects. *Horm Metab Res.* 2015;47(4):289–296. https://doi.org/10.1055/s-0034-1382011

3. Sabag A, Way KL, Keating SE, et al. Exercise and ectopic fat in type 2 diabetes: a systematic review and meta-analysis. Review. *Diabetes Metab.* 2017;43(3):195–210. https://doi.org/10.1016/j.diabet.2016.12.006. Epub February 2, 2017.

4. Borel AL, Nazare JA, Smith J, et al. Visceral and not subcutaneous abdominal adiposity reduction drives the benefits of a 1-year lifestyle modification program. Research support, non-US gov't. *Obesity (Silver Spring).* 2012;20(6):1223–1233. https://doi.org/10.1038/oby.2011.396

5. Gasmi A, Noor S, Menzel A, Doşa A, Pivina L, Bjørklund G. Obesity and insulin resistance: associations with chronic inflammation, genetic and epigenetic factors. *Curr Med Chem.* 2021;28(4):800–826. https://doi.org/10.2174/0929867327666200824112056

6. West CE, Renz H, Jenmalm MC, et al. The gut microbiota and inflammatory noncommunicable diseases: associations and potentials for gut microbiota therapies. *J Allergy Clin Immunol.* 2015;135(1):3–13. https://doi.org/10.1016/j.jaci.2014.11.012

7. Furman D, Campisi J, Verdin E, et al. Chronic inflammation in the etiology of disease across the life span. *Nat Med.* 2019;25(12):1822–1832. https://doi.org/10.1038/s41591-019-0675-0

8. Tsoupras A, Lordan R, Zabetakis I. Inflammation, not cholesterol, is a cause of chronic disease. *Nutrients.* 2018;10(5):604. https://doi.org/10.3390/nu10050604

9. Garcia-Bailo B, El-Sohemy A, Haddad PS, et al. Vitamins D, C, and E in the prevention of type 2 diabetes mellitus: modulation of inflammation and oxidative stress. *Biologics.* 2011;5:7–19. https://doi.org/10.2147/BTT.S14417

10. Lin CC, Tsweng GJ, Lee CF, Chen BH, Huang YL. Magnesium, zinc, and chromium levels in children, adolescents, and young adults with type 1 diabetes. *Clin Nutr. (Edinburgh).* 2016;35(4):880–884. https://doi.org/10.1016/j.clnu.2015.05.022

CHAPTER 3

1. Amati F, Dube JJ, Coen PM, Stefanovic-Racic M, Toledo FG, Goodpaster BH. Physical inactivity and obesity underlie the insulin resistance of aging. *Diabetes Care.* 2009;32(8):1547–1549. https://doi.org/10.2337/dc09-0267

2. Heir T, Erikssen J, Sandvik L. Life style and longevity among initially healthy middle-aged men: prospective cohort study. *BMC Public Health.* 2013;13:831. https://doi.org/10.1186/1471-2458-13-831

3. Marusic U, Narici M, Samanic B, Pisot R, Ritzmann R. Nonuniform loss of muscle strength and atrophy during bed rest: a systematic review. *J Appl Physiol (1985).* 2021;131(1):194–206. https://doi.org/10.1152/japplphysiol .00363.2020

4. Gillen JB, Estafanos S, Williamson E, et al. Interrupting prolonged sitting with repeated chair stands or short walks reduces postprandial insulinemia in healthy adults. *J Appl Physiol (1985).* 2021;130(1):104–113. https://doi.org /10.1152/japplphysiol.00796.2020

5. Kanaley JA, Colberg SR, Corcoran MH, et al. Exercise/physical activity in individuals with type 2 diabetes: a consensus statement from the American College of Sports Medicine. *Med Sci Sports Exerc.* 2022;54(2):353–368. https://doi.org/10.1249/mss.0000000000002800

6. Colberg SR, Sigal RJ, Yardley JE, et al. Physical activity/exercise and diabetes: a position statement of the American Diabetes Association. *Diabetes Care.* 2016;39(11):2065–2079. https://doi.org/10.2337/dc16 -1728

7. Eriksen L, Dahl-Petersen I, Haugaard SB, Dela F. Comparison of the effect of multiple short-duration with single long-duration exercise sessions on glucose homeostasis in type 2 diabetes mellitus. *Diabetologia.* 2007;50(11): 2245–2253. https://doi.org/10.1007/s00125-007-0783-0

8. Riddell MC, Gallen IW, Smart CE, et al. Exercise management in type 1 diabetes: a consensus statement. Review. *Lancet Diabetes Endocrinol.* 2017;5(5):377–390. https://doi.org/10.1016/S2213-8587(17)30014-1.

9. Khurshid S, Al-Alusi MA, Churchill TW, Guseh JS, Ellinor PT. Accelerometer-derived "weekend warrior" physical activity and incident cardiovascular disease. *JAMA.* 2023;330(3):247–252. https://doi.org/10 .1001/jama.2023.10875

10. Way KL, Hackett DA, Baker MK, Johnson NA. The effect of regular exercise on insulin sensitivity in type 2 diabetes mellitus: a systematic review and meta-analysis. *Diabetes Metab J.* 2016;40(4):253–271. https://doi.org/10 .4093/dmj.2016.40.4.253

288 • NOTES

11. Choi Y, Kim D, Kim SK. Effects of physical activity on body composition, muscle strength, and physical function in old age: bibliometric and meta-analyses. *Healthcare (Basel)*. 2024;12(2):197. https://doi.org/10.3390/healthcare12020197

12. Park SW, Goodpaster BH, Lee JS, et al. Excessive loss of skeletal muscle mass in older adults with type 2 diabetes. *Diabetes Care*. 2009;32(11):1993–1997. https://doi.org/dc09-0264:pii:10.2337/dc09-0264

13. Dunstan DW, Daly RM, Owen N, et al. Home-based resistance training is not sufficient to maintain improved glycemic control following supervised training in older individuals with type 2 diabetes. *Diabetes Care*. 2005;28(1):3–9. https://doi.org/ 10.2337/diacare.28.1.3:pii

14. Dunstan DW, Daly RM, Owen N, et al. High-intensity resistance training improves glycemic control in older patients with type 2 diabetes. *Diabetes Care*. 2002;25(10):1729–1736.https://doi.org/10.2337/diacare.25.10.1729

15. Taaffe DR, Duret C, Wheeler S, Marcus R. Once-weekly resistance exercise improves muscle strength and neuromuscular performance in older adults. *J Am Geriatr Soc*. 1999;47(10):1208–1214. https://doi.org/10.1111/j.1532-5415.1999.tb05201.x

16. Berger RA. Comparison of the effect of various weight training loads on strength. *Res Q*. 1965;36:141–146.

17. Liu Y, Ye W, Chen Q, Zhang Y, Kuo CH, Korivi M. Resistance exercise intensity is correlated with attenuation of HbA1c and insulin in patients with type 2 diabetes: a systematic review and meta-analysis. *Int J Environ Res Public Health*. 2019;16(1):140. https://doi.org/10.3390/ijerph16010140

18. Larkin ME, Barnie A, Braffett BH, et al. Musculoskeletal complications in type 1 diabetes. *Diabetes Care*. 2014;37(7):1863–1869. https://doi.org/10.2337/dc13-2361

19. Plastino M, Fava A, Carmela C, et al. Insulin resistance increases risk of carpal tunnel syndrome: a case-control study. *J Peripher Nerv Syst*. 2011;16(3):186–190. https://doi.org/10.1111/j.1529-8027.2011.00344.x

20. Ravindran Rajendran S, Bhansali A, Walia R, Dutta P, Bansal V, Shanmugasundar G. Prevalence and pattern of hand soft-tissue changes in type 2 diabetes mellitus. *Diabetes Metab*. 2011;37(4):312–317. https://doi.org/S1262-3636(10)00259-4:pii:10.1016/j.diabet.2010.09.008

21. Carapeto PV, Aguayo-Mazzucato C. Effects of exercise on cellular and tissue aging. *Aging (Albany)*. 2021;13:14522-14543. https://doi.org/10.18632/aging.203051

22. Piercy KL, Troiano RP, Ballard RM, et al. The physical activity guidelines for Americans. *JAMA*. 2018;320(19):2020–2028. https://doi.org/ 10.1001/jama.2018.14854

CHAPTER 4

1. Christovich A, Luo XM. Gut microbiota, leaky gut, and autoimmune diseases. *Front Immunol.* 2022;13:946248. https://doi.org/10.3389/fimmu.2022.946248
2. Martel J, Chang SH, Ko YF, Hwang TL, Young JD, Ojcius DM. Gut barrier disruption and chronic disease. *Trends Endocrinol Metab.* 2022;33(4):247–265. https://doi.org/10.1016/j.tem.2022.01.002
3. Fasano A. Zonulin and its regulation of intestinal barrier function: the biological door to inflammation, autoimmunity, and cancer. *Physiol Rev.* 2011;91(1):151–175. https://doi.org/10.1152/physrev.00003.2008
4. Mu Q, Kirby J, Reilly CM, Luo XM. Leaky gut as a danger signal for autoimmune diseases. *Front Immunol.* 2017;8:598. https://doi.org/10.3389/fimmu.2017.00598
5. Pasini E, Corsetti G, Assanelli D, et al. Effects of chronic exercise on gut microbiota and intestinal barrier in human with type 2 diabetes. *Minerva Med.* 2019;110(1):3–11. https://doi.org/10.23736/s0026-4806.18.05589-1
6. Qi Y, Goel R, Kim S, et al. Intestinal permeability biomarker zonulin is elevated in healthy aging. *J Am Med Dir Assoc.* 2017;18(9):810.e1–810.e4. https://doi.org/10.1016/j.jamda.2017.05.018
7. Ajala O, English P, Pinkney J. Systematic review and meta-analysis of different dietary approaches to the management of type 2 diabetes. *Am J Clin Nutr.* 2013;97(3):505–516. https://doi.org/10.3945/ajcn.112.042457
8. Rostgaard-Hansen AL, Esberg A, Dicksved J, et al. Temporal gut microbiota variability and association with dietary patterns: from the one-year observational DCH-NG MAX study. *Am J Clin Nutr.* 2024;119(4):1015–1026. https://doi.org/10.1016/j.ajcnut.2024.01.027
9. Wang G, Liu J, Xia Y, Ai L. Probiotics-based interventions for diabetes mellitus: a review. *Food Bioscience.* 2021;43:101172.
10. Naghshi S, Aune D, Beyene J, Mobarak S, Asadi M, Sadeghi O. Dietary intake and biomarkers of alpha linolenic acid and risk of all cause, cardiovascular, and cancer mortality: systematic review and dose-response meta-analysis of cohort studies. *BMJ.* 2021;375:n2213. https://doi.org/10.1136/bmj.n2213
11. Sundram K, Karupaiah T, Hayes KC. Stearic acid-rich interesterified fat and trans-rich fat raise the LDL/HDL ratio and plasma glucose relative to palm olein in humans. *Nutr Metab (London).* 2007;4(3). https://doi.org/10.1186/1743-7075-4-3

12. Lichtenstein AH. Dietary trans fatty acids and cardiovascular disease risk: past and present. *Curr Atheroscler Rep.* 2014;16(8):433. https://doi.org/10.1007/s11883-014-0433-1

13. Devries MC, Phillips SM. Creatine supplementation during resistance training in older adults—a meta-analysis. *Med Sci Sports Exerc.* 2014;46(6): 1194–1203. https://doi.org/10.1249/mss.0000000000000220

14. Livesey G, Taylor R, Livesey HF, et al. Dietary glycemic index and load and the risk of type 2 diabetes: a systematic review and updated meta-analyses of prospective cohort studies. Review. *Nutrients.* 2019;11(6):1280. https://doi.org/10.3390/nu11061280.

15. Weickert MO, Pfeiffer AFH. Impact of dietary fiber consumption on insulin resistance and the prevention of type 2 diabetes. *J Nutr.* 2018;148(1):7–12. https://doi.org/10.1093/jn/nxx008

16. Bell KJ, Fio CZ, Twigg S, et al. Amount and type of dietary fat, postprandial glycemia, and insulin requirements in type 1 diabetes: a randomized within-subject trial. *Diabetes Care.* 2020;43(1):59–66. https://doi.org/10.2337/dc19-0687

17. Bell KJ, Smart CE, Steil GM, Brand-Miller JC, King B, Wolpert HA. Impact of fat, protein, and glycemic index on postprandial glucose control in type 1 diabetes: implications for intensive diabetes management in the continuous glucose monitoring era. Review. *Diabetes Care.* 2015;38(6):1008–1015. https://doi.org/10.2337/dc15-0100

18. Zhao J, Stockwell T, Naimi T, Churchill S, Clay J, Sherk A. Association between daily alcohol intake and risk of all-cause mortality: a systematic review and meta-analyses. *JAMA Netw Open.* 2023;6(3):e236185. https://doi.org/10.1001/jamanetworkopen.2023.6185

19. Penumathsa SV, Maulik N. Resveratrol: a promising agent in promoting cardioprotection against coronary heart disease. *Can J Physiol Pharmacol.* 2009;87(4):275–286. httpsy09-013:pii:10.1139/Y09–013

20. Grober U, Reichrath J, Holick MF. Live longer with vitamin D? *Nutrients.* 2015;7(3):1871–1880. https://doi.org/10.3390/nu7031871

21. Raghuvanshi DS, Chakole S, Kumar M. Relationship between vitamins and diabetes. *Cureus.* 2023;15(3):e36815. https://doi.org/10.7759/cureus.36815

22. Lin CC, Huang YL. Chromium, zinc and magnesium status in type 1 diabetes. *Curr Opin Clin Nutr Metab Care.* 2015;18(6):588–592. https://doi.org/10.1097/MCO.0000000000000225

23. Adrogue HJ, Madias NE. The impact of sodium and potassium on hypertension risk. *Semin Nephrol.* 2014;34(3):257–272. https://doi.org/10.1016/j.semnephrol.2014.04.003

CHAPTER 5

1. Young EH, Pan S, Yap AG, Reveles KR, Bhakta K. Polypharmacy prevalence in older adults seen in United States physician offices from 2009 to 2016. *PLoS One.* 2021;16(8):e0255642. https://doi.org/10.1371/journal.pone.0255642

2. Fleck, A. More than half of Americans take prescribed meds daily. *Statista Consumer Insights.* 2023. Accessed August 1, 2024. https://www.statista.com/chart/31183/us-respondents-who-are-taking-prescribed-medicine.

3. Nicolussi S, Drewe J, Butterweck V, Meyer Zu Schwabedissen HE. Clinical relevance of St. John's wort drug interactions revisited. *Br J Pharmacol.* 2020;177(6):1212–1226. https://doi.org/10.1111/bph.14936

4. American Diabetes Association Professional Practice Committee. Cardiovascular disease and risk management: standards of care in diabetes—2024, part 10. *Diabetes Care.* 2024;47(suppl 1):S179–S218. https://doi.org/10.2337/dc24-S010

5. McCrimmon RJ, Henry RR. SGLT inhibitor adjunct therapy in type 1 diabetes. *Diabetologia.* 2018;61(10):2126–2133. https://doi.org/10.1007/s00125-018-4671-6

6. Snaith JR, Samocha-Bonet D, Evans J, et al. Insulin resistance in type 1 diabetes managed with metformin (INTIMET): study protocol of a double-blind placebo-controlled, randomised trial. *Diabet Med.* 2021;38:e14564. https://doi.org/10.1111/dme.14564

7. Handelsman Y, Henry RR, Bloomgarden ZT, et al. American Association of Clinical Endocrinologists and American College of Endocrinology Position Statement on the association of SGLT-2 inhibitors and diabetic ketoacidosis. *Endocr Pract.* 2016;22(6):753–762. https://doi.org/10.4158/EP161292.PS. Epub June 1, 2016.

8. Woo V, Connelly K, Lin P, McFarlane P. The role of sodium glucose cotransporter-2 (SGLT-2) inhibitors in heart failure and chronic kidney disease in type 2 diabetes. *Curr Med Res Opin.* 2019;35(7):1283–1295. https://doi.org/10.1080/03007995.2019.1576479. Epub February 15, 2019.

9. Joy NG, Tate DB, Davis SN. Counterregulatory responses to hypoglycemia differ between glimepiride and glyburide in nondiabetic individuals. *Metabolism.* 2015;64(6):729–737. https://doi.org/10.1016/j.metabol.2015.02.006

10. Want LL. Optimizing treatment success with an amylin analogue. *Diabetes Educ.* 2008;34(suppl 1):11S–7S. https://doi.org/34/1_suppl/11S: pii:10.1177/0145721707313940

292 • NOTES

11. Bajaj HS, Bergenstal RM, Christoffersen A, et al. Switching to once-weekly insulin icodec versus once-daily insulin glargine U100 in type 2 diabetes inadequately controlled on daily basal insulin: a phase 2 randomized controlled trial. *Diabetes Care*. 2021;44(7):1586–1594. https://doi.org /10.2337/dc20-2877

12. Aronson R, Li A, Brown RE, McGaugh S, Riddell MC. Flexible insulin therapy with a hybrid regimen of insulin degludec and continuous subcutaneous insulin infusion with pump suspension before exercise in physically active adults with type 1 diabetes (FIT Untethered): a single-centre, open-label, proof-of-concept, randomised crossover trial. *Lancet Diabetes Endocrinol*. 2020;8(6):511–523. https://doi.org/10.1016/s2213-8587 (20)30114-5

13. Karakuş KE, Yeşiltepe Mutlu G, Gökçe T, et al. Insulin requirements for basal and auto-correction insulin delivery in advanced hybrid closed-loop system: 4193 days' real-world data of children in two different age groups. *J Diabetes Sci Technol*. 2022:19322968221106194. https://doi.org/10.1177/193229 68221106194

14. Riddell MC, Turner LV, Patton SR. Is there an optimal time of day for exercise? A commentary on when to exercise for people living with type 1 or type 2 diabetes. *Diabetes Spectr*. 2023;36(2):146–150. https://doi.org /10.2337/dsi22-0017

15. Fabris C, Nass RM, Pinnata J, et al. The use of a smart bolus calculator informed by real-time insulin sensitivity assessments reduces postprandial hypoglycemia following an aerobic exercise session in individuals with type 1 diabetes. *Diabetes Care*. 2020;43(4):799–805. https://doi.org/10.2337 /dc19-1675

16. Morville T, Dohlmann TL, Kuhlman AB, et al. Aerobic exercise performance and muscle strength in statin users—the LIFESTAT study. *Med Sci Sports Exerc*. 2019;51(7):1429–1437. https://doi.org/10.1249/MSS.0000000000 001920.

17. de Oliveira LP, Vieira CP, Guerra FD, Almeida MS, Pimentel ER. Structural and biomechanical changes in the Achilles tendon after chronic treatment with statins. *Food Chem Toxicol*. 2015;77:50–57. https://doi.org/10.1016/j .fct.2014.12.014

18. Allen DC, Jedrzynski NA, Michelson JD, Blankstein M, Nelms NJ. The effect of dexamethasone on postoperative blood glucose in patients with type 2 diabetes mellitus undergoing total joint arthroplasty. *J Arthroplasty*. 2020; 35(3):671–674. https://doi.org/10.1016/j.arth.2019.10.030

NOTES • 293

CHAPTER 6

1. Look AHEAD Research Group. Eight-year weight losses with an intensive lifestyle intervention: the look AHEAD study. *Obesity (Silver Spring)*. 2014;22(1):5–13. https://doi.org/10.1002/oby.20662
2. North American Menopause Society. Menopause 101: a primer for the perimenopausal. Accessed August 1, 2024. https://www.menopause.org/for-women/menopauseflashes/menopause-symptoms-and-treatments/menopause-101-a-primer-for-the-perimenopausal
3. Ogawa M, Okamura M, Inoue T, Sato Y, Momosaki R, Maeda K. Relationship between nutritional status and clinical outcomes among older individuals using long-term care services: a systematic review and meta-analysis. *Clin Nutr ESPEN*. 2024;59:365–377. https://doi.org/10.1016/j.clnesp.2023.11.024
4. Adams KF, Leitzmann MF, Ballard-Barbash R, et al. Body mass and weight change in adults in relation to mortality risk. *Am J Epidemiol*. 2014;179(2):135–144. https://doi.org/10.1093/aje/kwt254
5. Kristensen SL, Rørth R, Jhund PS, et al. Cardiovascular, mortality, and kidney outcomes with GLP-1 receptor agonists in patients with type 2 diabetes: a systematic review and meta-analysis of cardiovascular outcome trials. *Lancet Diabetes Endocrinol*. 2019;7(10):776–785. https://doi.org/10.1016/s2213-8587(19)30249-9
6. Tsapas A, Karagiannis T, Kakotrichi P, et al. Comparative efficacy of glucose-lowering medications on body weight and blood pressure in patients with type 2 diabetes: a systematic review and network meta-analysis. *Diabetes Obes Metab*. 2021;23(9):2116–2124. https://doi.org/10.1111/dom.14451
7. Powell J, Taylor J. Use of dulaglutide, semaglutide, and tirzepatide in diabetes and weight management. *Clin Ther*. 2024;46:289–292. https://doi.org/10.1016/j.clinthera.2023.12.014
8. Wilding JPH, Batterham RL, Davies M, et al. Weight regain and cardiometabolic effects after withdrawal of semaglutide: the STEP 1 trial extension. *Diabetes Obes Metab*. 2022;24(8):1553–1564. https://doi.org/10.1111/dom.14725
9. Jadhav RA, Maiya GA, Hombali A, et al. Effect of physical activity promotion on adiponectin, leptin and other inflammatory markers in prediabetes: a systematic review and meta-analysis of randomized controlled trials. *Acta Diabetol*. 2021;58:419–429. https://doi.org/10.1007/s00592-020-01626-1
10. Fonseca VA, Capehorn MS, Garg SK, et al. Reductions in insulin resistance are mediated primarily via weight loss in subjects with type 2 diabetes on

semaglutide. *J Clin Endocrinol Metab*. 2019;104(9):4078–4086. https://doi .org/10.1210/jc.2018-02685

11. Landi F, Onder G, Gambassi G, Pedone C, Carbonin P, Bernabei R. Body mass index and mortality among hospitalized patients. *Arch Intern Med*. 2000;160(17):2641–2644. https://doi.org/10.1001/archinte.160.17.2641

12. Engin B, Willis SA, Malaikah S, et al. The effect of exercise training on adipose tissue insulin sensitivity: a systematic review and meta-analysis. *Obes Rev*. 2022:e13445. https://doi.org/10.1111/obr.13445

13. Kritchevsky SB, Beavers KM, Miller ME, et al. Intentional weight loss and all-cause mortality: a meta-analysis of randomized clinical trials. *PLoS One*. 2015;10(3):e0121993. https://doi.org/10.1371/journal.pone.0121993

14. Lv QB, Fu X, Jin HM, et al. The relationship between weight change and risk of hip fracture: meta-analysis of prospective studies. *Sci Rep*. 2015;5:16030. https://doi.org/10.1038/srep16030

15. Beavers KM, Neiberg RH, Houston DK, et al. Body weight dynamics following intentional weight loss and physical performance: the Look AHEAD movement and memory study. *Obes Sci Pract*. 2015;1(1):12–22. https://doi.org/10.1002/osp4.3

16. Cava E, Yeat NC, Mittendorfer B. Preserving healthy muscle during weight loss. *Adv Nutr*. 2017;8(3):511–519. https://doi.org/10.3945/an.116 .014506

17. Hall KD. Energy compensation and metabolic adaptation: "The Biggest Loser" study reinterpreted. *Obesity (Silver Spring)*. 2022;30(1):11–13. https://doi.org/10.1002/oby.23308

18. Frugé AD, Cases MG, Schildkraut JM, Demark-Wahnefried W. Associations between obesity, body fat distribution, weight loss and weight cycling on serum pesticide concentrations. *J Food Nutr Disord*. 2016;5(3). https://doi .org/10.4172/2324-9323.1000198

19. Visaria A, Setoguchi S. Body mass index and all-cause mortality in a 21st century U.S. population: a National Health Interview Survey analysis. *PLoS One*. 2023;18(7):e0287218. https://doi.org/10.1371/journal.pone .0287218

20. Hamman RF, Wing RR, Edelstein SL, et al. Effect of weight loss with lifestyle intervention on risk of diabetes. *Diabetes Care*. 2006;29(9):2102–2107. https://doi.org/29/9/2102:pii:10.2337/dc06-0560

21. Igudesman D, Crandell J, Corbin KD, et al. Weight management in young adults with type 1 diabetes: the advancing care for type 1 diabetes and obesity network sequential multiple assignment randomized trial pilot results. *Diabetes Obes Metab*. 2023;25(3):688–699. https://doi.org /10.1111/dom.14911

NOTES • 295

22. Zhu X, Zhang F, Chen J, et al. The effects of supervised exercise training on weight control and other metabolic outcomes in patients with type 2 diabetes: a meta-analysis. *Int J Sport Nutr Exerc Metab.* 2022:1–9. https://doi .org/10.1123/ijsnem.2021-0168

23. Graham HE, Madigan CD, Daley AJ. Is a small change approach for weight management effective? A systematic review and meta-analysis of randomized controlled trials. *Obes Rev.* 2022;23(2):e13357. https://doi.org/10.1111 /obr.13357

24. Kobayashi KM, Chan KT, Fuller-Thomson E. Diabetes among Asian Americans with BMI less than or equal to 23. *Diabetes Metab Syndr.* 2018;12(2): 169–173. https://doi.org/10.1016/j.dsx.2017.12.011

25. Mathew H, Farr OM, Mantzoros CS. Metabolic health and weight: understanding metabolically unhealthy normal weight or metabolically healthy obese patients. *Metabolism.* 2016;65(1):73–80. https://doi.org/10.1016/j .metabol.2015.10.019

26. Eckel N, Li Y, Kuxhaus O, Stefan N, Hu FB, Schulze MB. Transition from metabolic healthy to unhealthy phenotypes and association with cardiovascular disease risk across BMI categories in 90 257 women (the Nurses' Health Study): 30 year follow-up from a prospective cohort study. *Lancet Diabetes Endocrinol.* 2018;6(9):714–724. https://doi.org/10.1016/s2213 -8587(18)30137-2

27. An Q, Zhang QH, Wang Y, et al. Association between type 2 diabetes mellitus and body composition based on MRI fat fraction mapping. *Front Public Health.* 2024;12:1332346. https://doi.org/10.3389/fpubh.2024.1332346

28. Sabag A, Way KL, Keating SE, et al. Exercise and ectopic fat in type 2 diabetes: a systematic review and meta-analysis. Review. *Diabetes Metab.* 2017;43(3):195–210. https://doi.org/10.1016/j.diabet.2016.12.006

29. Beavers DP, Kritchevsky SB, Gill TM, et al. Elevated IL-6 and CRP levels are associated with incident self-reported major mobility disability: a pooled analysis of older adults with slow gait speed. *J Gerontol A Biol Sci Med Sci.* 2021;76(12):2293–2299. https://doi.org/10.1093/gerona/glab093

30. Wu J, Lin S, Chen W, et al. TNF-α contributes to sarcopenia through caspase-8/caspase-3/GSDME-mediated pyroptosis. *Cell Death Discov.* 2023;9(1):76. https://doi.org/10.1038/s41420-023-01365-6

31. Devries MC, Phillips SM. Creatine supplementation during resistance training in older adults—a meta-analysis. *Med Sci Sports Exerc.* 2014;46(6):1194–1203. https://doi.org/10.1249/mss.0000000000000220

32. Gualano B, De Salles Painneli V, Roschel H, et al. Creatine in type 2 diabetes: a randomized, double-blind, placebo-controlled trial. *Med Sci Sports Exerc.* 2011;43(5):770–778. https://doi.org/10.1249/MSS.0b013e3181fcee7d

296 • NOTES

CHAPTER 7

1. Biessels GJ, Despa F. Cognitive decline and dementia in diabetes mellitus: mechanisms and clinical implications. *Nat Rev Endocrinol.* 2018;14(10):591–604. https://doi.org/10.1038/s41574-018-0048-7
2. Zhou Y, Danbolt NC. Glutamate as a neurotransmitter in the healthy brain. *J Neural Transm (Vienna).* 2014;121(8):799–817. https://doi.org/10.1007/s00702-014-1180-8
3. Hassing L, Wahlin A, Winblad B, Bäckman L. Further evidence on the effects of vitamin B12 and folate levels on episodic memory functioning: a population-based study of healthy very old adults. *Biol Psychiatry.* 1999;45(11):1472–1480. https://doi.org/10.1016/s0006-3223(98)00234-0
4. Malone JI, Hanna S, Saporta S, et al. Hyperglycemia not hypoglycemia alters neuronal dendrites and impairs spatial memory. *Pediatr Diabetes.* 2008;9(6):531–539. https://doi.org/10.1111/j.1399-5448.2008.00431.x
5. Morley JE, Colberg SR. *The Science of Staying Young.* McGraw-Hill; 2007.
6. Pase MP. Modifiable vascular markers for cognitive decline and dementia: the importance of arterial aging and hemodynamic factors. *J Alzheimers Dis.* 2012;32(3):653–663. https://doi.org/10.3233/jad-2012-120565
7. National Institute on Aging. Thinking about your risk for Alzheimer's disease? five questions to consider. Accessed August 1, 2024. https://www.nia.nih.gov/health/alzheimers-causes-and-risk-factors/thinking-about-your-risk-alzheimers-disease-five
8. Gong CX, Grundke-Iqbal I, Iqbal K. Targeting tau protein in Alzheimer's disease. *Drugs Aging.* 2010;27(5):351–365. https://doi.org/10.2165/11536110-000000000-00000
9. Colberg SR, Somma CT, Sechrist SR. Physical activity participation may offset some of the negative impact of diabetes on cognitive function. *J Am Med Dir Assoc.* 2008;9(6):434–438. https://doi.org/S1525-8610(08)00121-7:pii:10.1016/j.jamda.2008.03.014
10. Zhang R, Liu S, Mousavi SM. Cognitive dysfunction and exercise: from epigenetic to genetic molecular mechanisms. *Mol Neurobiol.* 2024. https://doi.org/10.1007/s12035-024-03970-7
11. Centers for Disease Control and Prevention. Diabetes and mental health. Accessed August 1, 2024. https://www.cdc.gov/diabetes/managing/mental-health.html
12. Franquez RT, de Souza IM, Bergamaschi CC. Interventions for depression and anxiety among people with diabetes mellitus: review of systematic

reviews. *PLoS One.* 2023;18(2):e0281376. https://doi.org/10.1371/journal.pone.0281376

13. Albert PR. Why is depression more prevalent in women? *J Psychiatry Neurosci.* 2015;40:219–221. https://doi.org/10.1503/jpn.150205

14. Flygare O, Boberg J, Rück C, et al. Association of anxiety or depression with risk of recurrent cardiovascular events and death after myocardial infarction: a nationwide registry study. *Int J Cardiol.* 2023;381:120–127. https://doi.org/10.1016/j.ijcard.2023.04.023

15. Hankerson SH, Weissman MM. Church-based health programs for mental disorders among African Americans: a review. *Psychiatr Serv.* 2012;63(3):243–249. https://doi.org/10.1176/appi.ps.201100216

16. Apaydin EA, Maher AR, Shanman R, et al. A systematic review of St. John's wort for major depressive disorder. *Syst Rev.* 2016;5(1):148. https://doi.org/10.1186/s13643-016-0325-2

17. Harvard University Study of Adult Development. Harvard second generation study. Accessed August 1, 2024. https://www.adultdevelopmentstudy.org/

CHAPTER 8

1. Giannos P, Prokopidis K, Candow DG, et al. Shorter sleep duration is associated with greater visceral fat mass in US adults: findings from NHANES, 2011–2014. *Sleep Med.* 2023;105:78–84. https://doi.org/10.1016/j.sleep.2023.03.013

2. Kanagasabai T, Riddell MC, Ardern CI. Inflammation, oxidative stress, and antioxidant micronutrients as mediators of the relationship between sleep, insulin sensitivity, and glycosylated hemoglobin. *Front Public Health.* 2022;10:888331. https://doi.org/10.3389/fpubh.2022.888331

3. Amaral FGD, Cipolla-Neto J. A brief review about melatonin, a pineal hormone. *Arch Endocrinol Metab.* 2018;62:472–479. https://doi.org/10.20945/2359-3997000000066

4. Vinik AI. The conductor of the autonomic orchestra. *Front Endocrinol (Lausanne).* 2012;3:71. https://doi.org/10.3389/fendo.2012.00071

5. Brown JJ, Colberg SR, Baskette K, Pribesh SG, Vinik AI. Impact of melatonin supplementation on autonomic nervous system function in adults with type 2 diabetes: a pilot study. *Acta Sci.* 2021;2:7–16. https://www.actascientific.com/ASCR/pdf/ASCR-02-0173.pdf

298 • NOTES

6. Morrissey EC, Casey B, Dinneen SF, Lowry M, Byrne M. Diabetes distress in adolescents and young adults living with type 1 diabetes. *Can J Diabetes.* 2020; 44:537–540. https://doi.org/10.1016/j.jcjd.2020.03.001
7. Centers for Disease Control and Prevention. 10 tips for coping with diabetes distress. Accessed August 1, 2024. https://www.cdc.gov/diabetes/managing /diabetes-distress/ten-tips-coping-diabetes-distress.html.
8. Klaperski S, Koch E, Hewel D, Schempp A, Müller J. Optimizing mental health benefits of exercise: the influence of the exercise environment on acute stress levels and wellbeing. *Mental Health & Prevention.* 2019;15:200173.

CHAPTER 9

1. US Preventive Services. Final recommendation statement: colorectal cancer: screening. Accessed August 1, 2024. https://www.uspreventiveservicestaskforce .org/uspstf/recommendation/colorectal-cancer-screening
2. Gao P, Zhang X, Yin S, et al. Meta-analysis of the effect of different exercise mode on carotid atherosclerosis. *Int J Environ Res Public Health.* 2023;20:2189. https://doi.org/10.3390/ijerph20032189
3. Arnett DK, Blumenthal RS, Albert MA, et al. 2019 ACC/AHA guideline on the primary prevention of cardiovascular disease: a report of the American College of Cardiology/American Heart Association Task Force on Clinical Practice Guidelines. *J Am Coll Cardiol.* 2019;74:e177–e232. https://doi.org /10.1016/j.jacc.2019.03.010
4. He W, Fang T, Fu X, Lao M, Xiao X. Risk factors and the CCTA application in patients with vulnerable coronary plaque in type 2 diabetes: a retrospective study. *BMC Cardiovasc Disord.* 2024;24(1):89. https://doi.org/10.1186 /s12872-024-03717-1
5. Wilkins JT, Ning H, Stone NJ, et al. Coronary heart disease risks associated with high levels of HDL cholesterol. *J Am Heart Assoc.* 2014;3(2):e000519. https://doi.org/10.1161/jaha.113.000519
6. Englund EK, Langham MC, Wehrli FW, et al. Impact of supervised exercise on skeletal muscle blood flow and vascular function measured with MRI in patients with peripheral artery disease. *Am J Physiol Heart Circ Physiol.* 2022;323(3):H388–H396. https://doi.org/10.1152/ajpheart.00633.2021
7. Lievre MM, Moulin P, Thivolet C, et al. Detection of silent myocardial ischemia in asymptomatic patients with diabetes: results of a randomized trial and meta-analysis assessing the effectiveness of systematic screening. *Trials.* 2011;12:23. https://doi.org/1745-6215-12-23:pii:10.1186/1745-6215-12-23

NOTES • 299

8. Abudawood M. Diabetes and cancer: a comprehensive review. *J Res Med Sci.* 2019;24:94. https://doi.org/10.4103/jrms.JRMS_242_19

9. Rawla P. Epidemiology of prostate cancer. *World J Oncol.* 2019;10(2):63–89. https://doi.org/10.14740/wjon1191

10. Barsouk A, Padala SA, Vakiti A, et al. Epidemiology, staging and management of prostate cancer. *Med Sci (Basel).* 2020;8:28. https://doi.org/10.3390/medsci8030028

11. American Cancer Society. Signs and symptoms of cancer. Accessed August 1, 2024. https://www.cancer.org/cancer/diagnosis-staging/signs-and-symptoms-of-cancer.html

12. Centers for Disease Control and Prevention. Oral health fast facts: diabetes. Accessed August 1, 2024. https://www.cdc.gov/oralhealth/fast-facts/diabetes/index.html

13. Stöhr J, Barbaresko J, Neuenschwander M, Schlesinger S. Bidirectional association between periodontal disease and diabetes mellitus: a systematic review and meta-analysis of cohort studies. *Sci Rep.* 2021;11(1):13686. https://doi.org/10.1038/s41598-021-93062-6

14. Song TJ, Chang Y, Jeon J, Kim J. Oral health and longitudinal changes in fasting glucose levels: a nationwide cohort study. *PLoS One.* 2021;16(6): e0253769. https://doi.org/10.1371/journal.pone.0253769

CHAPTER 10

1. Yang Y, Hu X, Zhang Q, Zou R. Diabetes mellitus and risk of falls in older adults: a systematic review and meta-analysis. *Age Ageing.* 2016;45(6):761–767. https://doi.org/10.1093/ageing/afw140

2. American Diabetes Association Professional Practice Committee. Older adults: standards of care in diabetes—2024, part 13. *Diabetes Care.* 2024;47(suppl 1):S244–S257. https://doi.org/10.2337/dc24-S013

3. Centers for Disease Control and Prevention. Older adult fall prevention. Accessed August 1, 2024. https://www.cdc.gov/falls/index.html

4. Fan Y, Wei F, Lang Y, Liu Y. Diabetes mellitus and risk of hip fractures: a meta-analysis. *Osteoporos Int.* 2016;27(1):219–228. https://doi.org/10.1007/s00198-015-3279-7

5. Handsaker JC, Brown SJ, Bowling FL, Marple-Horvat DE, Boulton AJ, Reeves ND. People with diabetic peripheral neuropathy display a decreased stepping accuracy during walking: potential implications for risk of tripping. *Diabet Med.* 2016;33(5):644–649. https://doi.org/10.1111/dme.12851

300 • NOTES

6. Poggiogalle E, Lubrano C, Gnessi L, et al. The decline in muscle strength and muscle quality in relation to metabolic derangements in adult women with obesity. *Clin Nutr.* 2019;38(5):2430–2435. https://doi.org/10.1016/j .clnu.2019.01.028. Epub February 10, 2019.

7. Marcos-Pérez D, Sánchez-Flores M, Proietti S, et al. Association of inflammatory mediators with frailty status in older adults: results from a systematic review and meta-analysis. *Geroscience.* 2020;42(6):1451–1473. https://doi .org/10.1007/s11357-020-00247-4

8. Centers for Disease Control and Prevention. Osteoporosis or low bone mass in older adults: United States, 2017–2018. Accessed August 1, 2024. https:// www.cdc.gov/nchs/products/databriefs/db405.htm

9. Pouresmaeili F, Kamalidehghan B, Kamarehei M, Goh YM. A comprehensive overview on osteoporosis and its risk factors. *Ther Clin Risk Manag.* 2018;14: 2029–2049. https://doi.org/10.2147/tcrm.s138000

10. Management of osteoporosis in postmenopausal women: the 2021 position statement of the North American Menopause Society. *Menopause.* 2021;28(9):973–997. https://doi.org/10.1097/gme.0000000000001831

11. Hu Y, Li X, Yan X, Huang G, Dai R, Zhou Z. Bone mineral density spectrum in individuals with type 1 diabetes, latent autoimmune diabetes in adults, and type 2 diabetes. *Diabetes Metab Res Rev.* 2021;37(3):e3390. https://doi.org /10.1002/dmrr.3390

12. Paulin TK, Malmgren L, McGuigan FE, Akesson KE. Osteosarcopenia: prevalence and 10-year fracture and mortality risk—a longitudinal, population-based study of 75-year-old women. *Calcif Tissue Int.* 2024; 114:315–325. https://doi.org/10.1007/s00223-023-01181-1

13. Guo D, Zhao M, Xu W, He H, Li B, Hou T. Dietary interventions for better management of osteoporosis: an overview. *Crit Rev Food Sci Nutr.* 2021;63(1):125–144. https://doi.org/10.1080/10408398.2021.1944975

14. Tai V, Leung W, Grey A, Reid IR, Bolland MJ. Calcium intake and bone mineral density: systematic review and meta-analysis. *BMJ.* 2015;351:h4183. https://doi.org/10.1136/bmj.h4183

15. Manoj P, Derwin R, George S. What is the impact of daily oral supplementation of vitamin D3 (cholecalciferol) plus calcium on the incidence of hip fracture in older people? A systematic review and meta-analysis. *Int J Older People Nurs.* 2023;18(1):e12492. https://doi.org/10.1111 /opn.12492

16. Vorland CJ, Stremke ER, Moorthi RN, Hill Gallant KM. Effects of excessive dietary phosphorus intake on bone health. *Curr Osteoporos Rep.* 2017;15(5):473–482. https://doi.org/10.1007/s11914-017-0398-4

17. Levin VA, Jiang X, Kagan R. Estrogen therapy for osteoporosis in the modern era. *Osteoporos Int.* 2018;29(5):1049–1055. https://doi.org/10.1007/s00198-018-4414-z

18. Centers for Disease Control and Prevention. Arthritis. Accessed August 1, 2024. https://www.cdc.gov/chronicdisease/resources/publications/factsheets/arthritis.htm

19. Cheng YJ, Imperatore G, Caspersen CJ, Gregg EW, Albright AL, Helmick CG. Prevalence of diagnosed arthritis and arthritis-attributable activity limitation among adults with and without diagnosed diabetes: United States, 2008–2010. *Diabetes Care.* 2012;35(8):1686–1691. https://doi.org/10.2337/dc12-0046

20. Abate M, Schiavone C, Salini V, Andia I. Management of limited joint mobility in diabetic patients. *Diabetes Metab Syndr Obes.* 2013;6:197–207. https://doi.org/10.2147/dmso.s33943

21. Kraus VB, Sprow K, Powell KE, et al. Effects of physical activity in knee and hip osteoarthritis: a systematic umbrella review. *Med Sci Sports Exerc.* 2019;51(6):1324–1339. https://doi.org/10.1249/mss.0000000000001944

22. Howes MJ, Simmonds MS. The role of phytochemicals as micronutrients in health and disease. *Curr Opin Clin Nutr Metab Care.* 2014;17(6):558–566. https://doi.org/10.1097/mco.0000000000000115

23. Wandel S, Juni P, Tendal B, et al. Effects of glucosamine, chondroitin, or placebo in patients with osteoarthritis of hip or knee: network meta-analysis. *BMJ.* 2010;341:c4675. https://doi.org/10.1136/bmj.c4675

APPENDIX A

Resistance Exercises

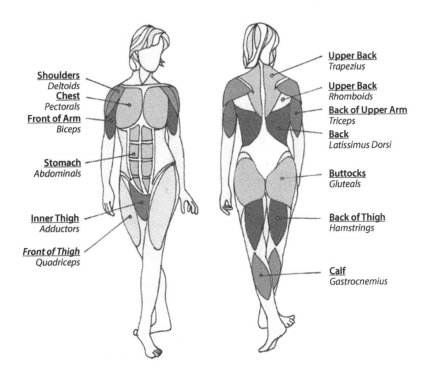

UPPER-BODY EXERCISES

1. Chest press

Main muscles worked: deltoids (front section), pectorals, triceps

Directions:

- Lie down on your back, holding a dumbbell in each hand right above your chest with your elbows bent. If you're using a resistance band, position the band underneath your shoulders, and grab onto it with your hands.

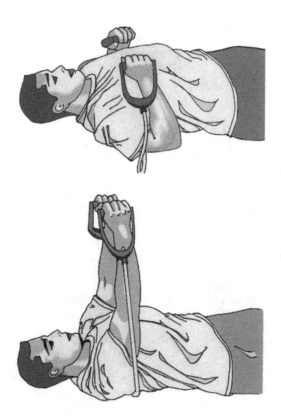

- Push both arms up in the air until they are almost straight, shoulder-width apart, and hold this position for several seconds.
- Bring your arms back down to your sides until your elbows touch the mat, allowing the dumbbells (or resistance band) to return to the starting position.

2. Shoulder press

Main muscles worked: deltoids (anterior and middle portion), trapezius muscles, triceps

Directions:

- In a sitting position, hold the dumbbells right above your shoulders with bent elbows, or if using a resistance band, sit on it, and hold the band on either side at shoulder height.

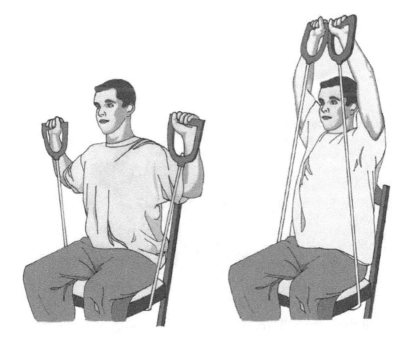

- Keep your abdominal muscles tight and your torso straight.
- Push up until your arms are almost straight and the dumbbells or your hands come close to meeting in the middle above your head.
- Slowly return to the starting position.

3. Lateral arm raise

Main muscles worked: deltoids (middle and back sections), trapezius muscles

Directions:

- Sit with your back straight and the dumbbells in your hands at your sides or the resistance band underneath your bottom.
- If using the resistance band, grasp one end of it in each hand, and clench your fists with your knuckles facing upward.

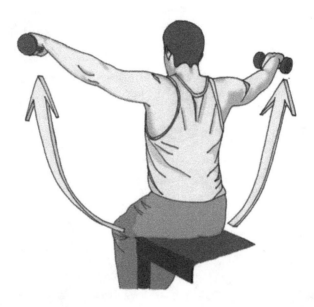

- Lift the dumbbells (or pull the resistance band up and straight out to the side) until both arms are level with your shoulders, keeping your elbows slightly bent.
- Hold this position for a few seconds before slowly returning to the starting position.
- Relax your neck and try not to hunch your shoulders to ensure that your shoulder and neck muscles are doing the work (not your arms).

4. Modified push-ups

Main muscles worked: pectorals, deltoids (anterior portion), triceps

Directions:

- Get on your hands and knees on the floor or mat.
- If using a band for extra resistance, position it across your back, and hold one end of it in each hand so that it is somewhat tight when your elbows are straight.
- Place your hands shoulder-width apart on the mat.

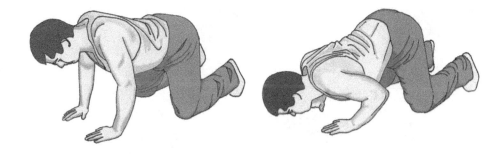

- Tighten your abdominal muscles to straighten your lower back, and lower yourself (from your knees, not your feet) down toward the mat as far as possible without touching it.
- Push yourself back up until your arms are extended but without locking your elbows.
- If this exercise is too hard, stand facing a wall, and place your arms on it at shoulder height and your feet about a foot away; then, do your push-ups off the wall (with or without a resistance band).

5. Double-arm row

Main muscles worked: deltoids (back portion), latissimus dorsi, rhomboids, biceps

Directions:

- Stand with your feet in line with your hips with a dumbbell in each hand.
- If using a resistance band, position it underneath your feet, and hold the band with both hands at your sides.
- With your knees slightly bent, bend your upper body forward from the hips about 70 degrees.
- Straighten your arms so that your palms face each other.
- Pull the dumbbells or resistance band in toward your waist so that your elbows move up past your hips, but keep your upper arms close to your sides.

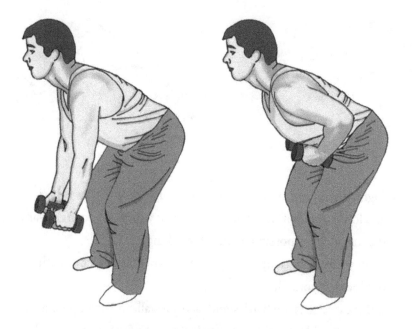

- Alternately, sit with your legs out in front of you (knees slightly bent) and the resistance band wrapped around the soles of both feet. Then, keeping your torso straight, pull your arms straight back, keeping your arms by your sides during the movement.

6. Lat pull-down

Main muscles worked: latissimus dorsi, biceps

Directions:

- Sit with your back straight, and hold both ends of the resistance band, one in each hand.
- Still grasping the band, fully extend your arms above your head.
- With your arms still extended, stretch the band so that both hands go out to the sides slightly wider than your shoulders, and hold this position for a few seconds.

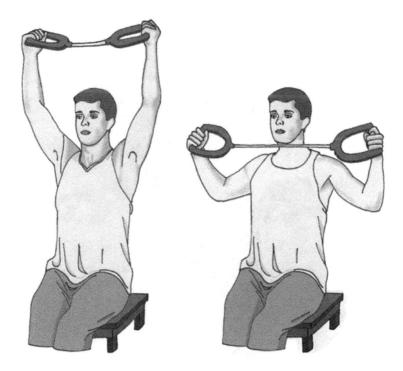

- Pull the stretched band down toward your chin, pulling it out by bending at the elbow to stretch it further.
- Squeeze your shoulder blades together, and feel the muscles in your back, shoulders, and arms contract.
- Hold this position for a few seconds and then extend your arms back up above your head, allowing the band to relax.

7. Biceps curls

Main muscles worked: biceps

Directions:

- Sit down holding the dumbbells, and drop both arms to your sides so that your elbows are in line with your hips with your palms facing forward.

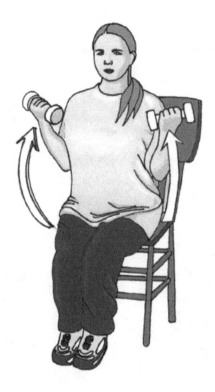

- Bring your knees and feet together, keeping your stomach muscles tight to support your lower back.
- Lift the dumbbells, bending your elbows while keeping your upper arms stationary at your sides until the dumbbells almost touch your chest.
- Slowly return the dumbbells to the starting position.
- Alternatively, do one arm at a time by supporting the elbow of the arm holding the dumbbell against the inside of your knee on the same side.
- With resistance bands, secure one end of the band under your right foot, and grasp the other end in your right hand, palm face up. Complete the same movement, keeping your upper arm close to your torso at all times. Switch sides to work the left arm.

UPPER-BODY EXERCISES 311

8. Triceps curls

Main muscles worked: triceps

Directions:

- Sit on the bench or chair holding one dumbbell in your lap with both hands.
- Lift the dumbbell straight up until your arms are straight and the dumbbell is directly overhead.
- Bend your arms at the elbows only, and lower the dumbbell behind your head.
- Keep your stomach muscles tight throughout the movement to support your lower back and keep it straight.
- Lift the dumbbell straight overhead again by straightening your arms at the elbow to return to the starting position.

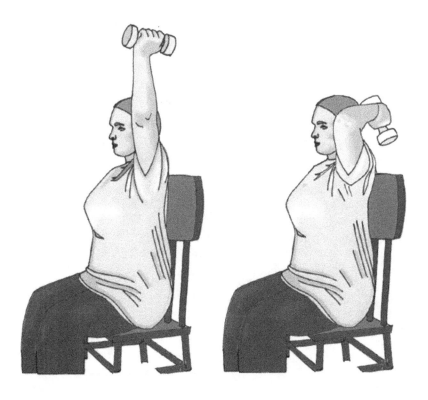

- If using a resistance band, hold it in your right hand while you raise your right arm with your elbow bent, and drop the band straight down behind your back on the right side. Then grab the other end in your left hand by reaching behind across the small of your back. Alternatively, straighten and bend at the elbow (with your upper arm still raised at the shoulder) and then switch the positioning of your arms to work the left side.

9. Chair push-ups

Main muscles worked: deltoids, triceps

Directions:

- Using your arms (not your legs), grasp the arms of a sturdy chair.

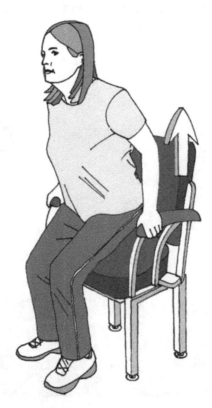

- Slowly push your body as far as you can up off the chair, hold your weight, and slowly lower yourself back down.
- Alternately, lean slightly forward while doing the push-up, or you can start by sitting on a phone book or cushion.

LOWER-BODY EXERCISES

1. One-leg press
Main muscles worked: quadriceps, gluteus, calves

Directions:

- Sit on the floor with your legs out in front of you and your knees slightly bent.
- Hold one end of the resistance band in each hand, and place it around the sole of your left foot with your left knee fully bent.
- Straighten your left leg (without locking your knee) while pulling on both sides of the resistance band.
- Continue to pull against the resistance band as you return your knee to the bent position.

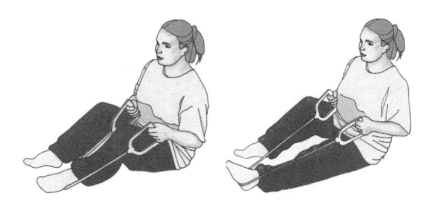

- Repeat the exercise with your right leg.
- Alternatively, tie the resistance band in a circle around the leg of a chair, then sit on the chair, place the sole of your foot inside the other end of the band, and straighten your leg almost fully.

2. Squats

Main muscles worked: quadriceps, hamstrings, gluteus, calves

Directions:

- Stand with a dumbbell in each hand and your feet shoulder-width apart, with your toes pointing slightly out to each side.
- If you're using a resistance band, tie both ends of your band onto a straight bar or broom handle, which is then placed squarely across your shoulders with you standing on the loop of the tied band.

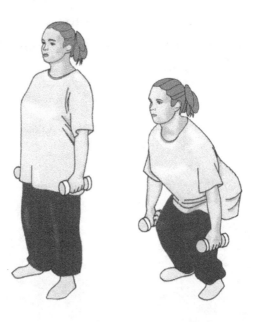

- Keep your body weight over the back portion of your foot rather than your toes; if needed, lift your arms out in front of you to shoulder height to stay balanced.
- Begin squatting down but stop before your thighs are parallel to the floor (at about a 70-degree bend), keeping your back flat and your abdominal muscles firm at all times.
- Hold that position for a few seconds before pushing up from your legs until your body is upright in the starting position.
- Do squats with your back against a smooth wall if needed to maintain your balance.

3. Knee dips

Main muscles worked: quadriceps, hamstrings, gluteus, calves

Directions:

- Get into a sprinter's position, facing forward as though you were at the starting line of a race, with one leg forward and one behind and your hands on the floor in front of you.
- Bend both legs as much as is comfortable, bringing your knees as close to the floor as possible without touching.
- Push your body upward until your legs are almost straight without locking your knees.

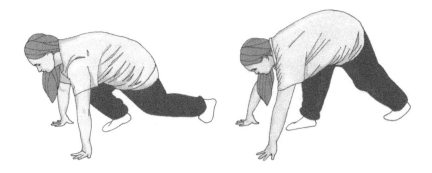

- Switch the position of your legs and repeat.
- Lunge variation: if you prefer, you can perform essentially the same exercise by standing up and starting with your legs spaced the same way, knees straight, and then bend your back knee to bring both knees closer to the floor while maintaining your balance.

4. Knee lift

Main muscles worked: quadriceps, hip flexors, abdominals

Directions:

- Lie on your back with your knees bent.
- Bend at your hip until your bent knees are positioned straight up over your hips at a 90° angle.
- Tighten your abdominals to hold your lower back flat against the floor.
- Lift your head slightly off the floor, and position the resistance band across the front of your thighs, just above the knees.
- Holding the band in your hands, stretch it by pulling your hands out more to the sides.
- Pull your knees in toward your chest against the band to increase the resistance against your lower abdominals and the front of your thighs.

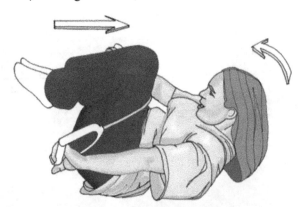

- Slowly return to the starting position.
- If holding your head slightly off the floor is too hard, relax your neck muscles and rest your head on the floor.

5. Seated leg extensions

Main muscles worked: quadriceps

Directions:

- Sit on the chair with your back straight and your feet and knees shoulder width apart.
- If using additional resistance, place the band around the bottom of your right foot with your knee bent (or use the ankle weight), and then place your foot back on the floor.
- Holding both ends of the band in your right hand or without any extra resistance, slowly straighten your right knee, and lift your foot (without moving at your hip) until your leg is straight out in front of you (at a 90-degree angle to your torso).

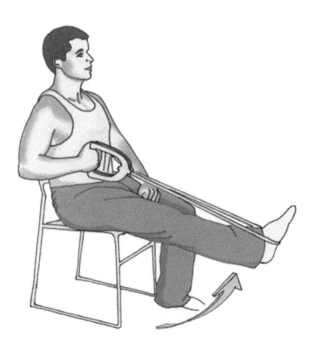

318 • APPENDICES AND RESOURCES

- Slowly bend your right knee, and return to the starting position.
- Repeat with the left leg.

6. Standing leg curls

Main muscles worked: hamstrings

Directions:

- Stand with your hands more than shoulder-width apart against a wall or other support and bend your right knee.
- Keeping your knees close together, smoothly lift your right heel up toward your bottom.
- Hold your heel as close to your bottom as you can, and lift it for several seconds before returning your foot slowly to the floor.

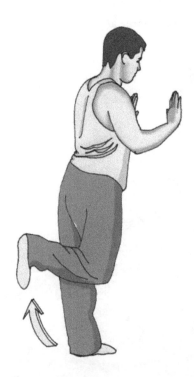

- To increase the intensity of the curl, place a resistance band around your right ankle with your knee bent, and hold both ends of it with your right hand during the movement.
- Repeat with the left leg.

7. Standing side leg raises

Main muscles worked: gluteus, outer thighs

Directions:

- Stand behind a chair and hold on to the back, or place your hands shoulder-width apart on the wall.
- Lift your right leg straight out to the side until your foot is about 6–12 inches off the floor and hold for several seconds.
- Keep your torso erect throughout the movement, and slightly bend the leg that is supporting your weight.

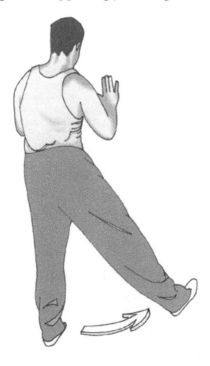

- Return your leg to the starting position.
- For added resistance, tie your resistance band into a circle, and place it around both of your ankles before lifting one leg at a time out as far as you can against the band.
- Repeat with your left leg.

8. Calf raises

Main muscles worked: calves

Directions:

- Stand erect with the balls of your feet on a stable, elevated surface (stair or ledge).
- If using dumbbells, hold a dumbbell in one or both hands.
- Keeping your body straight, balance on the ball of your foot, and lift your heels as high as possible for several seconds.

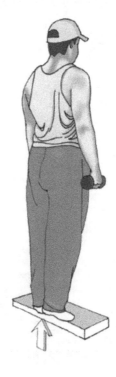

- Slowly lower your heels down as far as possible (even past being level with the stair or ledge, if you can).
- Alternately, work one calf at a time with or without holding a dumbbell.

9. Sit-to-stand

Main muscles worked: abdominals, thighs

Directions:

- Sit toward the front of a sturdy chair and fold your arms across your chest.
- Keep your back and shoulders straight while you lean forward slightly, and practice using only your legs to stand up slowly and to sit back down.
- To assist you initially, place pillows on the chair behind your lower back.

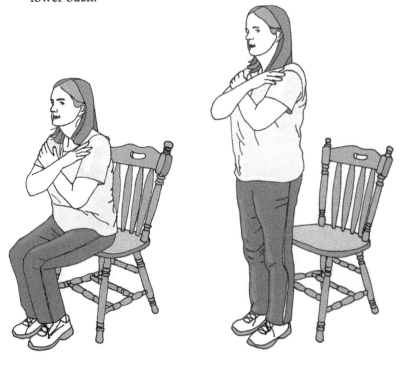

LOWER-BACK AND ABDOMINAL EXERCISES

1. Crunches

Main muscles worked: abdominals

Directions:

- Lie down on your back with your knees bent.
- Place your hands on your head right behind your ears.
- While breathing out, contract your abdominal muscles to lift your head, neck, and shoulders off the floor and curl forward no more than 45 degrees.
- Hold for a moment before returning to the starting position, then repeat.
- You can also do these sitting upright in a chair (see chair sit-ups).

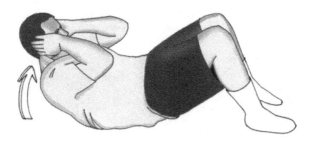

2. Waist worker

Main muscles worked: abdominals (obliques)

Directions:

- Lie on your back on the mat with your legs bent, your feet flat on the floor, and your left hand behind your head.

- Stretch your right hand across your body toward your opposite (left) knee, and circle your hand three times around your knee in a counterclockwise direction; your right shoulder blade will lift off the mat.
- Repeat the circular movement around the right knee using your left arm but in a clockwise motion.
- Keep your head in a neutral position, and relax your neck to ensure the contraction is in your abdominal area only.

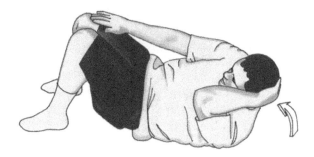

3. Chair sit-ups

Main muscles worked: lower back

Directions:

- Sit up straight in a chair with your feet on the floor and your hands to your sides for support.
- Bend forward, keeping your lower back as straight as possible, and move your chest down toward your thighs.
- Slowly straighten back up, using your lower-back muscles to raise your torso.

- For added resistance, put a resistance band under both feet before you start and hold one end in each hand during the movement.

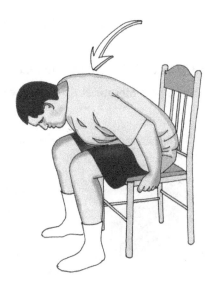

4. Lower-back strengthener

Main muscles worked: lower back, gluteus

Directions:

- Lie on your stomach with your arms straight over your head and your chin resting on the floor between your arms.
- Keeping your arms and legs straight, simultaneously lift your feet and your hands as high off the floor as possible (aim for at least three inches off the floor.
- Hold that position (sort of a Superman flying position) for 10 seconds if possible, and then allow your arms and legs to relax back onto the floor.
- If this exercise is too difficult to start, try lifting just your legs or arms off the floor separately—or even just one limb at a time.

LOWER-BACK AND ABDOMINAL EXERCISES 325

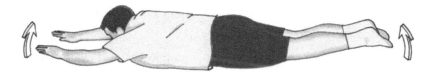

5. Pelvic tilt

Main muscles worked: lower back, lower abdominals

Directions:

- Lie on your back on the floor with your knees bent, feet flat on the floor and hands either by your sides or supporting your head.
- Firmly tighten your bottom, forcing your lower back flat against the floor.
- Relax and repeat.

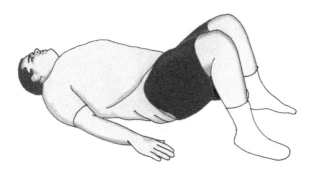

6. Suitcase lift (or, the proper way to lift items)

Main muscles worked: lower back, lower body (muscles involved in squats)

Directions:

- After placing the dumbbells or household items slightly forward and between your feet on the floor, stand in an upright position with your back straight.

326 • APPENDICES AND RESOURCES

- Keep your arms straight, with your hands in front of your abdomen.
- With your back straight, bend only your knees, and reach down to pick up the dumbbells.
- Pick up the dumbbells or items in both hands, then push up with your legs and stand upright, keeping your back straight.

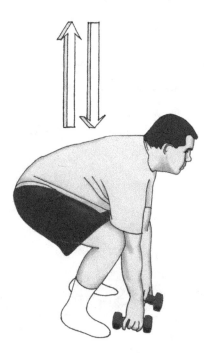

7. Planks and plank variations

Main muscles worked: core body muscles, abdominals, lower back, gluteus, quadriceps, trapezius, deltoids, forearms, calves, and so on.

An alternate exercise to work on your abdomen, lower back, buttocks, thighs, upper arms, neck, shoulders, and lower calves all at the same time is any type of plank (not pictured):

- It's possible to do basic planks propped up on your forearms, high planks with your arms straight, modified planks from your

LOWER-BACK AND ABDOMINAL EXERCISES 327

knees (instead of your toes), single-arm or single-leg planks, side planks, side plank crunches or leg lifts, walking planks, and other variations.

- Just search "plank exercises" or "plank variations" online to find plenty of illustrations and instructions to perform as many types of planks as your heart desires.
- This is admittedly a tough exercise, but try to work up to holding each plank for 30–60 seconds, rest, and repeat until you're too fatigued to do any more.

APPENDIX B

Stretches

UPPER-BODY STRETCHES

1. Neck stretch

Directions:

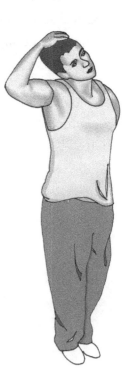

- Stand with your feet apart and your knees slightly bent, or sit in a chair with your back straight and your feet on the floor.
- Relax your shoulders and gently bend your head toward your right shoulder.
- For an extra stretch, reach up with your right hand, and apply a gentle pressure against the left side of your head in the direction of the stretch.
- Repeat on the left side.
- In addition, stretch your neck by tipping your head forward toward your chest and backward toward your spine.

2. Shoulder/upper-back stretch

Directions:

- Stand with your feet a little apart, your knees slightly bent, and your stomach muscles slightly tensed.
- Relax your shoulders and pull your right arm horizontally across your chest by grabbing onto your elbow with your left hand.
- Repeat with your left arm.
- You can alternately do this exercise while seated in a chair.

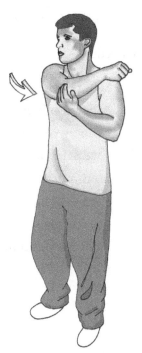

3. Chest/shoulder stretch

Directions:

- If standing, bend your knees slightly, tense your stomach muscles, and relax your shoulders.
- If seated, sit forward in your chair to make room for your arms to go behind you.
- Cross your hands behind your back, and concentrate on bringing your shoulder blades toward each other as far as you can.

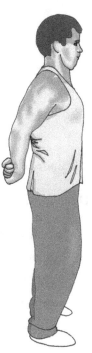

4. Shoulder/biceps stretch

Directions:

- Sit on the floor with both legs extended out in front of you and your knees bent.
- Keeping your back straight, put your hands behind you with your palms flat on the floor and your fingers pointing away from your body.
- With your hands stationary, scoot your bottom forward until you feel the stretch in your shoulders.
- Hold this position.

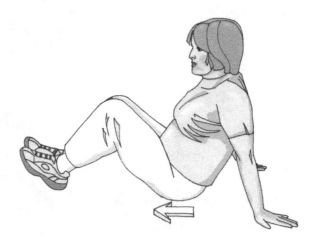

5. Upper-back/triceps stretch

Directions:

- Sitting or standing, grab your right elbow with your left hand and push it straight up and back until the upper portion of your right arm is next to your right ear.
- Keep your spine and neck as straight as possible during this movement.
- Repeat this stretch with your left arm.

UPPER-BODY STRETCHES 331

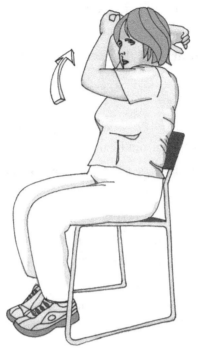

6. Wrist stretch

Directions:

- Press your hands together with your elbows down.
- Raise your elbows as nearly parallel to the floor as possible while keeping your hands together in a prayer position.
- Hold and then repeat.

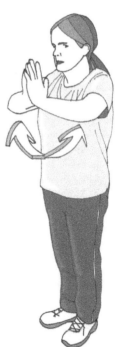

LOWER-BODY STRETCHES

1. Quadriceps (front of thigh) stretch

Directions:

- Holding onto a chair or the wall with your left hand, grab your right ankle with your right hand by bending at the knee, and bring your heel as close as you can toward your bottom (touching it, if possible).
- If that stretch is easy for you, take it one step further by leaning forward slightly from that position and pulling your heel up and about six inches away from your bottom.
- Repeat with the other leg.
- You can also do this stretch by lying on your side and stretching the leg on top.

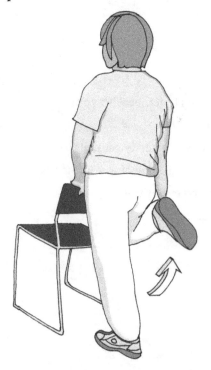

2. Hamstring (back of thigh) stretch

Directions:

- Sitting on the floor with your back straight, place your legs in a V.
- Next, bend your right knee, and bring your foot in toward your groin area.
- Gently lean out over your left leg to stretch the back of your left thigh (don't worry if you aren't able to lean very far).
- Repeat with the other leg.
- Reminder: never bend your knee outward in the opposite direction (even though you may see other people doing so) to avoid injury to the knee joint.

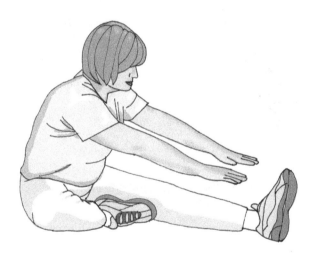

3. Alternate hamstring (back of thigh) stretch

Directions:

- Stand behind a chair with your legs straight.
- Hold the back of the chair with both hands.

- Bend forward from your hips, not from your waist, keeping your entire back and shoulders straight until your upper body is parallel to the floor.
- Hold this position, relax, and repeat.

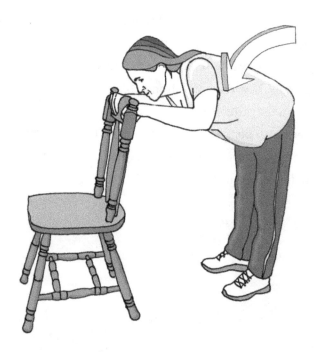

4. Gluteal (bottom) stretch

Directions:

- Lie on your back with both knees bent and your feet flat on the floor.
- Grab both your knees with your hands and pull them up toward your chest as far as you can.

- Hold this position for several seconds before releasing.
- You can also do this stretch using one leg at a time.

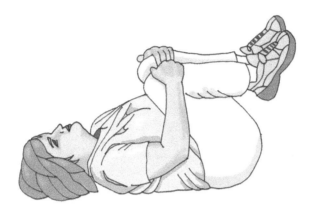

5. Calf stretch

Directions:

- With straight arms, put your hands on a wall in front of you, and place your feet shoulder-width apart.
- Move your left foot back about twelve inches more while bending your right knee.
- Holding your back and your left knee straight, bend your elbows slightly and lean in a few inches toward the wall to stretch your left calf.
- Then, keeping your foot flat on the ground, slightly bend your left knee for an even greater stretch.
- Repeat this exercise with the other leg.

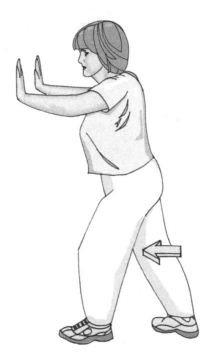

6. Ankle stretch

Directions:

- With your shoes off, sit toward the front end of a chair and lean back, using pillows to support your back.
- Slide your feet away from the chair and in front of you to stretch out your legs.
- With your heels still on the floor, point your toes away from you until you feel a stretch in the front part of your ankles and hold the position.
- If you don't feel a stretch, lift your heels slightly off the floor while doing this stretch.

LOWER-BODY STRETCHES 337

- For a different stretch, try pointing your toes to the left and the right in addition to forward, and roll each foot around at the ankle in circles going clockwise and then in reverse (which will also help improve your balance).

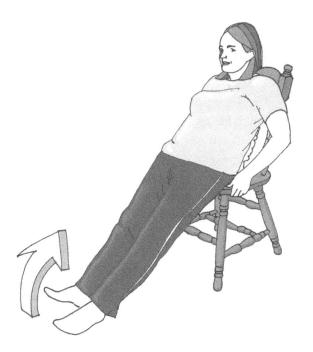

338 • APPENDICES AND RESOURCES

OTHER STRETCHES

1. Abdominal stretch

Directions:

- Lie down on your front with your arms over your head.
- Pull your arms in until you are propped up on your elbows.
- Gently arch your neck backward as far as is comfortable toward your bottom, keeping your hips on the floor.
- Hold the stretch for several seconds.

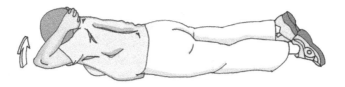

2. Back/gluteal stretch

Directions:

- Lie down on your back with your arms straight out from your sides.
- Bend your right knee and then stretch it across your left leg while trying to keep your right hip on the ground.
- Repeat with the other leg.

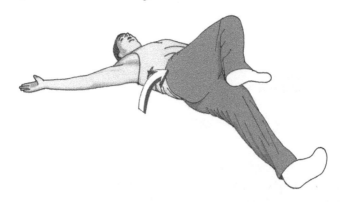

3. Complete back (cat) stretch

Directions:

- Kneel on all fours, keeping your knees in line with your hips, your hands in line with your shoulders, and everything in line with your spine, which should be flat.
- Breathe in as you slowly arch your back toward the ceiling with your abs tight, your pelvis tilted, and your gaze toward your navel.
- Breathe out as you reverse the action, drawing your chest toward the floor.

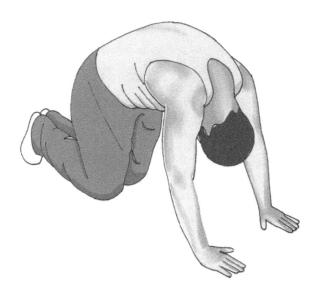

4. Total body stretch

Directions:

- Lie on your back with your legs together, and extend your arms straight up over your head to lie on the floor.
- Tighten your abs and press your lower back firmly to the floor.

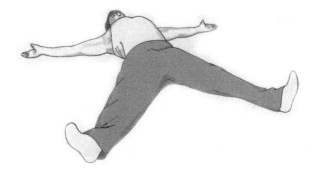

- Take a deep breath in, and as you breathe out, extend both your arms and legs as far away from your body and out to the sides as you can.
- Hold for several seconds before returning to the starting position.

> **APPENDIX C**

Beers List of Drugs to Be Avoided over Age 65 (2023)

Beers criteria category	Drug or drug class example	Concern
Analgesics	Meperidine	Neurotoxicity, delirium
Antibiotics	Ciprofloxacin with warfarin	Increased bleeding
Antiseizure	Carbamazepine	Syndrome of inappropriate antidiuretic hormone secretion (SIADH)
Antidepressants	Duloxetine	Nausea, diarrhea
Antigout	Colchicine	Bone marrow toxicity
Antihistamines	Brompheniramine	Confusion, cognitive impairment, delirium, falls
Antihypertensives	Alpha-blockers	Hypotension
Antiplatelets or anticoagulants	Edoxaban	Renal impairment
Antipsychotics	Any antipsychotic	Stroke, cognitive decline, delirium
Anxiolytics	Benzodiazepines	Impaired metabolism, cognitive impairment, unsteady gait
Cardiac	Disopyramide	Heart failure
Central nervous system	Dimenhydrinate	Confusion, cognitive impairment, delirium
Diabetes	Chlorpropamide	Hypoglycemia
Gastrointestinal	H_2 antagonist for delirium	Worsening delirium
Hormones	Estrogen	Breast cancer, endometrial cancer
Hypnotics	Barbiturates	Dependence, overdose
Musculoskeletal	Muscle relaxers	Confusion, dry mouth, constipation
NSAIDs	Aspirin (more than 325 mg/day)	Ulcer, gastrointestinal bleeding or perforation
Respiratory	Atropine	Confusion, cognitive impairment, delirium
Urinary	Desmopressin	Low sodium in blood (hyponatremia)
Vasodilators	Ergoloid mesylates	Lack of intended results

APPENDIX D

Precautions about Potential Drug Interactions

Taking certain medications when you have other conditions can actually worsen your health. Our best advice is the following:

- For chronic constipation, avoid the use of calcium channel antagonists, imipramine, amitriptyline, and doxepin (the last three are antidepressants).
- If you have seizures, don't take Wellbutrin (also an antidepressant).
- If you have high blood pressure, avoid taking any medications with pseudoephedrine, which can be found in many over-the-counter decongestants such as Sudafed.
- If you have peptic ulcer disease, avoid aspirin and other nonsteroidal anti-inflammatory drugs, such as ibuprofen (Nuprin, Advil) and Naproxen (Aleve).
- If you have Parkinson's disease, avoid Reglan and many antipsychotic drugs.
- If you have hyponatremia (low levels of sodium in your blood, below 135 mEq/L), don't take Paxil, Zoloft, Luvox, or Celexa as they could make it even worse.

Resources (Online)

American Cancer Society
- cancer.org

American Diabetes Association
- diabetes.org

American Heart Association
- americanheart.org

American Institute for Cancer Research
- aicr.org

American Society of Clinical Oncology
- cancer.net

American Society on Aging
- asaging.org

American Stroke Association
- stroke.org

Association of Diabetes Care & Education Specialists
- adces.org

Centers for Disease Control and Prevention
- Still Going Strong
- cdc.gov/still-going-strong

Dr. Sheri Colberg's websites—exercise and diabetes information
- shericolberg.com
- diabetesmotion.com
- dmacademy.com (Diabetes Motion Academy)

Johns Hopkins Medicine—Diabetes Self Management Patient Education Materials

- hopkinsmedicine.org/general-internal-medicine/core-resources/patient-handouts

Joslin Diabetes Center, Beth Israel Lahey Health

- joslin.org

Living With Diabetes

- cdc.gov/diabetes/living-with

National Cancer Institute

- cancer.gov

National Coalition for Cancer Survivorship

- canceradvocacy.org

National Council on Aging

- ncoa.org/older-adults

Prevent Cancer Foundation

- preventcancer.org

Taking Control of Your Diabetes

- tcoyd.org

U.S. Department of Health and Human Services

- Diabetes Evidence-Based Resources
- health.gov/healthypeople/objectives-and-data/browse-objectives/diabetes/evidence-based-resources
- Healthy Aging
- hhs.gov/aging/healthy-aging/index.html

U.S. Food and Drug Administration—Advice about Eating Fish

- fda.gov/food/consumers/advice-about-eating-fish

Index

acanthosis nigricans, 41

ACE inhibitors, 171

acetaminophen, 277–78

acetylcholine, 196–97

adiponectin, 132, 178

adrenaline, 33, 81

aerobic activities, 62, 65, 66–72, 90, 91, 100, 106, 241–42

aging, 3–5, 7–8, 12, 56, 57, 59, 90–91, 100–101, 173, 264–65; positive attitude toward, 5, 6–7, 62, 213–14, 216, 259, 283; premature, 90, 107, 119, 121

AIDS/HIV, 33, 193, 200

alcohol consumption, 6, 52, 112, 134, 136, 145, 184, 207–8, 234, 235, 249, 262; adverse health effects, 52, 135, 249, 250, 262, 267–68; beneficial health effects, 110–11, 134–35, 143

allergies/allergic reactions, 33, 50, 142, 145, 146

alpha-glucosidase inhibitors, 154, 155

alpha-lipoic and alpha-linoleic acid, 120–21, 122, 142

Alzheimer's disease, 9–10, 59, 61, 122, 134–35, 195, 196, 197, 198, 199, 200–201, 202, 203–4, 255, 263

amino acids, 18, 120–21

amylin, 158, 159

andropause, 52, 173

anemia, 28, 139, 157, 180, 191, 200, 262–63, 264–65, 266

angiotensin II receptor blockers, 171

anthocyanins, 119–20, 135

anticoagulants (blood thinners), 136, 171, 243, 278, 342

antidepressants, 171, 193, 200, 207

antihistamines, 151, 222, 341

anti-inflammatory agents, 92–93, 95, 102, 132, 277–80

antioxidants, 54, 55, 112, 117, 119–20, 135, 220, 233, 239, 271, 279

antiplatelet medications, 243

anxiety, 32, 48, 52, 61, 142, 194, 195, 227, 266; memory impairment effects, 195, 198–99, 200–201, 228

A1C (glycated hemoglobin), 22–25, 27–28, 35, 235–36, 254

appetite, 252, 253; enhancers, 192, 193; factors affecting, 18–19, 23–24, 146, 172, 176, 189–91, 264–65

arteries, plaque-related blockage, 125, 240, 241–42, 243

arthritis: post-traumatic, 275; psoriatic, 274, 275; rheumatoid, 191–92, 255, 274, 275, 279. *See also* osteoarthritis

aspirin, 125, 152, 243, 278

asthma, 16, 33, 50, 73, 108–9, 137, 140, 164

atrial fibrillation, 243, 263

autoimmune diseases, 49, 107, 108–9, 137

balance, 6, 9, 81, 247, 261, 262–65; exercises/training, 6, 56, 66, 77, 82–85, 100, 106, 262, 266; test for, 82

benfotiamine, 139–40

beta-amyloid protein, 203–4

beta-blockers, 32, 69, 170

beta-carotene, 55

beta cells, 18, 19, 20, 22, 40, 44, 49, 156, 159

biguanides, 154, 155, 158

bisphosphonates, 273

bladder cancer, 248, 251, 252

blood cancers, 255

blood fats, 127, 140, 239, 240. *See also* cholesterol; triglycerides

346 • INDEX

blood flow, 59, 61, 67, 90, 105, 126, 242; to brain, 59, 105, 202, 203, 243; to heart, 134, 170, 240, 245, 246–47

blood glucose, 13–14, 39–40, 42–43, 61

blood glucose level monitoring, 17, 33–37; continuous and intermittent (CGM) systems, 35–36; finger-stick glucose meters, 17, 33–34

blood glucose levels: in diabetes diagnostic testing, 22–25; effect of physical activity on, 70, 81, 154; effect of weight loss on, 176; fluctuations, 32, 33, 42; in prediabetes, 20, 21–22; tight range, 27. *See also* monitoring, of blood glucose levels

blood glucose levels, high. *See* hyperglycemia

blood glucose levels, low *See* hypoglycemia

blood glucose management, 9, 10, 12–37, 233; balanced approach, 10, 13, 15, 16, 32, 281; personalized targets and goals in, 13, 14–15, 25–28, 29, 37, 65, 281; self-care tips for, 12, 13

blood pressure, 25, 58, 61, 140, 141, 233, 236, 244, 245. *See also* hypertension; hypotension

blood sugar. *See* blood glucose

blood tests, for diabetes (or prediabetes), 22–25

body composition, 188–89

body fat, 11, 18, 31–32, 52, 53, 67, 174; adverse health effects, 176, 177, 178, 239, 249–50; assessment, 184–89; beneficial functions, 176–77, 178; cells, 20, 39, 42, 43, 46–47, 49, 161; medication and toxin accumulation in, 149, 172, 180

body fat distribution, 9–10, 21; visceral/abdominal, 46–47, 52, 177, 178, 183–88, 265

body mass index (BMI), 179, 181, 184, 185–86, 188–89

body temperature regulation (thermoregulation), 101, 177

body weight, 171, 172–93; assessment, 184–89, 236; exercises, 62, 75–76; gain, 6, 52, 172–73, 176–77, 181, 278–79; healthy/"just right," 6, 63, 181–84, 207–8, 230, 236, 250, 282; implication for insulin therapy, 41

body weight loss, 6, 130, 155, 158, 175–76, 181–82, 233; health benefits of, 21, 31–32, 43, 44–45, 47, 172, 176, 233, 234, 277; reversible causes, 189–90; unhealthy/unintentional, 16, 23–24, 52, 156, 159, 175–76, 177–80, 189–93, 206, 252, 264; weight regain after, 179–80, 182–83

bone marrow transplantation, 251

bone mass/density, 58, 61, 75, 229, 230, 266–73; loss, 9–10, 91, 96, 97, 206–7; maintenance, 138, 140, 259, 267–73, 283; measurement/scans, 6, 94, 189, 268. *See also* osteopenia; osteoporosis

brain: aging-related changes, 59, 199; benefits of physical activity on, 59, 61, 105, 201; benefits of sleep for, 215–17, 218, 219; blood flow to, 59, 105, 202, 203, 243; brain-stimulating exercises, 210–13, 265, 266; glucose utilization in, 14, 42; growth factors, 201; hypoglycemia effects, 29; insulin content, 204; neurofibrillary tangles, 203–4; tumors, 200–201. *See also* cognitive impairment

breast cancer, 6, 58, 135, 249, 251, 252

caffeine, 47, 138, 145, 235, 272

calcium, 117, 138, 141, 268–71, 272

calcium-channel blockers, 171

calories, 61, 116, 128–29, 133–34, 136–37, 173, 182

cancer, 7, 50, 108–9, 114, 177–78, 206, 230, 247–48, 247–54, 249; diabetes

INDEX · 347

management in, 16; metastatic, 248–49; prevention/risk reduction, 11, 58, 61, 121, 122, 132, 230, 231, 232, 234, 235, 236, 247, 249–51, 283; risk factors, 9–10, 125, 248, 255; screenings/early detection, 234, 236, 237–38, 251; treatment, 4, 237, 248–49, 251–54. See also *specific types of cancer*

canes, 6, 56, 262, 263, 277

carbohydrates, 64, 111, 128–34, 138–39, 175, 182; carbohydrate-to-insulin ratio, 133–34; digestion and metabolism, 129, 132, 136, 153, 154, 162; effect on blood glucose levels, 14, 42, 45, 70, 124, 127, 128, 129–32, 134, 162, 168; glycemic index and load, 129–32, 162; rapid-acting, 30–31; refined (simple), 53, 124–25, 132, 183; storage in muscles, 45, 61, 63, 65

cardiovascular diseases (CVDs), 8, 29, 50, 54, 231, 262–63, 265; as Alzheimer's disease risk factor, 204; implication for exercise participation, 88; insulin resistance and, 43; management, 238–47; as mortality cause, 7, 114, 177, 230, 238, 239–40, 245, 247; prevention/risk reduction, 11, 58, 61, 62, 67, 70, 114, 125, 127, 135, 230, 231, 232, 233–34, 239, 245, 281, 283; risk factors, 9–10, 22, 26, 125–26, 138, 180, 187–88, 204, 219, 239, 241, 242, 255; treatment, 149–50, 170

caregivers and caregiving, 8–9, 195–96

carpal tunnel syndrome, 85

cervical cancer, 249, 251

chest pain, 68, 72, 73, 87, 89, 90, 170, 239, 246–47

chocolate and cacao, 119, 125, 140

cholesterol: food content, 124–25, 271; HDL, 25, 134, 236, 241–42; LDL, 168, 169, 180, 236, 240, 241–42

cholesterol, elevated levels, 32, 50, 53, 88–89, 124, 147–48, 265; management, 32, 39, 40, 61, 114, 115–16, 126, 130, 140, 149–50, 168–69, 236, 239, 241–42, 281

chondroitin, 279–80

chromium, 141

chronic diseases, 3–4, 50, 147–48; diabetes as risk for, 231; multiple co-occurring, 149–50; prevention and control, 232–38

chronic obstructive pulmonary disease, 50, 89, 90, 234

circadian rhythm, 219–20, 221, 224

Cleveland, Gerald, 213–14

coffee, 47, 119, 125

cognitive ability, 11, 59, 105, 208–14, 219

cognitive behavioral therapy, 206

cognitive impairment, 35, 195–97; mild, 198–99, 261; risk factors, 9–10, 29–30, 187–88, 194, 222, 243, 247, 264. See also memory loss

cola sodas, 138, 235, 272

Colberg, Sheri, 1–3; *The Athlete's Guide to Diabetes*, 167; *The Science of Staying Young*, 208–9

collagen, 85

colorectal cancer, 6, 58, 237–38, 247–48, 251; prevention, 114, 115–16, 232, 236, 237–38, 249, 250, 251

constipation, 52, 252; prevention and management, 114, 117, 136, 142, 232, 235; risk factors, 114, 191, 206, 271, 341, 342

corticosteroids (steroids; glucocorticoids), 16, 24, 32, 51, 171, 193, 278–79

corticotrophic-releasing factor, 206

cortisol, 42, 48, 49, 184, 206–7, 222–23, 225, 229, 278

COVID-19, 6, 7, 51, 174, 189, 236

C-reactive protein (CRP), 51, 127
creatine supplements, 127, 128, 192
cycling, 67, 68, 69, 75, 90, 98, 102, 105,
    277; stationary, 62, 68, 72, 88, 90, 98
cytokines, 50–51, 176, 191–92, 241,
    265

decongestants, 152
dehydration, 28, 71, 73, 101, 114, 156,
    170, 184–85, 188–89
dementia, 9–10, 29, 30, 194–95, 197,
    198, 199, 263; differentiated from
    mild cognitive impairment, 201–3;
    prevention and management, 11, 59,
    142, 187–88, 202–3; types, 202
dental health, 190, 191, 231, 235,
    254–57, 283
depression, 191, 195, 202, 204–8;
    causes/risk factors, 52, 108–9, 140,
    205–7, 219, 225; memory impair-
    ment effects, 198–99, 200–201, 228;
    treatment/management, 32, 59, 61,
    147–48, 152, 171, 194, 207–8, 229,
    266, 283
dextrose. See glucose
diabetes management, 9–10, 233;
    balanced approach, 10, 13, 15, 16; as
    "diabetes distress" cause, 225–28;
    heterogeneity in, 8–9; step-based
    approach, 10–11, 281–84. See also
    blood glucose management; goals/
    targets, in diabetes management
diabetes medications: cost, 225, 227.
    See also glucose-lowering medi-
    cations; insulin therapy; names of
    specific medications
diabetes medications, injectable
    (non-insulin), 158–59
diabetes medications, oral. See glucose-
    lowering medications
diabetes mellitus, definition, 17; gesta-
    tional, 18, 35; lipoatrophic, 176, 178;
    medications-induced, 18; as mortality

cause, 114; onset age, 8; types of,
    17–22. See also prediabetes; type 1
    diabetes; type 2 diabetes
diabetes supplies, 227
diabetic ketoacidosis, 156
diagnosis, of diabetes, 22–25; impact on
    health status, 40; insulin resistance
    diagnosis and, 41; prediabetes, 22–25
diarrhea, 73, 191, 253
diet/food, 16; advanced glycation end
    products, 132; anti-inflammatory, 53,
    54–55, 239; anti-inflammatory prop-
    erties, 55; for bone health, 268–72;
    for cancer prevention, 234, 249, 250;
    for cardiovascular health, 234, 239,
    240; fast food, 54, 110, 126–27; for
    frailty prevention, 265; glucose con-
    tent, 14; glycemic index and load,
    129–32, 162; for gum health, 256; for
    gut health, 110–43; for hyperglyce-
    mia management, 31; as inflamma-
    tion cause, 49; for insulin resistance
    management, 43, 47; for joint pain
    management, 279; low-carbohydrate,
    111, 115, 129; low-fat, 124; medicinal
    activity, 110; Mediterranean, 110–11;
    as osteoporosis cause, 267–68;
    Paleo, 116; plant-based, 55, 113, 114,
    117–21, 128, 143, 271; processed/
    refined, 53, 54, 111, 113–14, 126–27,
    132, 139, 183, 233, 234, 250; role in
    Alzheimer's disease, 203; trends and
    fads, 175; vegan, 129, 139; for weight
    loss and maintenance, 132, 175,
    182–83, 233. See also diet; eating
    habits; meals
disabilities, 9, 100
disaccharides, 14
diuretics, 32, 170, 245–46; potassium-
    sparing, 170
dizziness and vertigo, 29, 68, 72, 73, 88,
    142, 170, 222, 247, 261, 262–63, 266
DNA, 53, 119, 120, 140, 248

dopamine, 132, 196–97
DPP-4 inhibitors (gliptins), 154, 155, 156, 158, 159
dual-energy X-ray absorptiometry (DEXA) scans, 188–89

eating habits, 11, 233, 252; before bedtime, 221; for body weight maintenance, 189–90; during cancer treatment, 253; for constipation prevention, 232; effect on insulin resistance, 22, 44; for insulin production, 21; for muscle mass increase/maintenance, 16, 172
edema, 157, 245
end-of-life care, 149
endorphins, 196–97, 229
endurance: aging-related decrease, 90–91; muscular strength *versus*, 79; physical activity/exercise-related enhancement, 61, 63, 83, 100, 104, 106. *See also* aerobic activities
epicondylitis (golfer's or tennis elbow), 85, 87, 102
erectile dysfunction, 206, 231
esophageal cancer, 250
estrogen, 52, 173, 272
exercise. *See* physical activity/exercise
exercise stress testing, 88–89
eye exercises, 103
eye problems. *See* vision impairment/ eye disorders

falls, 150, 258–63, 259–60; prevention, 6, 56, 61, 77, 83, 85, 100, 230, 261–63, 283; risk factors, 9, 16–17, 27, 29, 32, 258, 260–61, 262
fasting: blood glucose levels during/ after, 14, 32, 254; intermittent, 183–84; nighttime, 47; plasma glucose test, 22, 23, 24, 25, 41, 235
fat, dietary, 111, 121–26, 125–26, 128–29, 134, 234, 249, 271

fatigue, 29, 64, 142, 150; causes, 23–24, 51, 58, 81, 140, 169, 225, 246, 252–53, 262; memory impairment effects, 198–99
fatty acids, 18
feet: daily checking of, 72; diabetes-related symptoms, 88; exercise-related blisters/injuries, 72, 73, 93, 95; flexibility exercises, 85; plantar fasciitis, 93; role in prevention of falls, 262
fiber, dietary, 47, 53, 111, 113–17, 128, 130, 133, 233, 235, 256
fight or flight response, 48–49, 184, 226
flavones, flavonoids, flavonols, 119, 125, 135
flexibility/stretching exercises, 66, 85–87, 91, 96, 97, 100, 106, 261–62, 266, 328–40; lower-body, 332–37; upper-body, 328–31
fluid intake, 71, 73, 112, 117, 136, 235; water intoxication and, 71
fractures, 27, 29, 61, 95, 97, 138, 177, 180, 189, 258, 259–60, 263, 264, 267
frailty, 9–10, 29, 177, 190, 258, 259, 264–66, 265–66, 280, 283
free radicals, 52, 53, 54, 119
fructose (fruit sugar), 13–14, 54, 131, 132–33

GABA, 196–97
galactose, 13–14
gastroparesis, 154, 191
genetic factors, 4; in Alzheimer's disease, 203; in BMI, 185; in body fat distribution, 188; in cancer, 237, 249, 251; in diabetes, 19, 20, 231; in disease, 231, 238; in drug interactions, 149; in hypertension, 244–45; in longevity, 5, 8, 42; in muscle fiber type, 63–64; in osteoporosis, 267
geriatricians, 150
GIP hormone, 156, 159, 175

352 • INDEX

insulin sensitizers, 204
insulin therapy, 152–53; adverse health
effects, 29; aerobic exercise and, 70;
automated insulin delivery (AID, or
hybrid closed-loop) system, 37; basal
insulins, 161–62, 166; bolus (mealtime) insulins, 133–34, 162–63, 164,
166, 167; carbohydrate-to-insulin
ratio, 133–34; cost, 227; dosage, 43,
160, 162–63, 164, 167; duration of
activity, 160, 161, 166; formulations,
160, 161–63; as hypoglycemia risk,
30, 31, 151; insulin analogues, 160;
insulin-delivery systems, 37, 38–39,
160, 161–62, 163–64; insulin inhal-
ers, 160, 164; insulin patch "pumps,"
164; insulin pen needles, 163; insulin
pumps, 160, 161–62, 164, 166; as
insulin resistance risk, 41; insulin
syringes, 163; onset time, 160, 161,
162, 166, 167; peak of activity, 160,
161, 162; physical activity/exercise
and, 70, 102–3, 154, 164–68; in type
1 diabetes, 160
interleukin-6, 191–92
interstitial fluids, 35
iron, dietary intake, 117
irritable bowel syndrome, 109

joints, 3, 40; arthritic, 60, 142,
274–80; benefits of sleep for, 60;
body weight-related stress, 178;
diabetes-related problems, 97;
"frozen," 85, 97, 275; inflexibility,
59; injuries, 67, 275; limiting conditions, 85–86; maintenance, 259;
pain in, 60, 61, 67, 68, 69, 71, 77,
81, 88, 90, 141, 224, 276, 277–80;
physical activity/exercise effects,
60, 61, 80, 81, 85–87.229, 234;
replacement, 80
Joslin Geriatric Diabetes Program, 1,
204

ketoacidosis, diabetic, 156
kidneys: cancer, 255; disease, 28, 29,
43, 71, 88–89, 95–96, 140, 149–50;
effect of hyperglycemia on, 26; effect
of medications on, 149, 153, 157,
178
knee: arthritis, 275, 277; injuries, 96,
102; pain, 76–77; replacement, 280

lactic acid, 64
lactose, 14
leptin, 178
libido (sex drive), 61, 206
lifespan/longevity, 5, 7; factors
affecting, 7–8, 57, 61, 122–23, 135,
174–75, 230, 264, 281
lifestyle: impact on aging process, 3; as
type 2 diabetes cause, 20
lifestyle changes, health-beneficial, 2,
22, 53–55; for diabetes management,
10, 38, 39, 40, 44
ligaments, 93, 169, 229, 274, 276
liver: advanced glycation end products
and, 132; cancer, 248; cholesterol
production in, 124; drug metabolism/
damage in, 149, 153, 277–78; excess
body fat storage in, 46–47, 54, 180,
187; fatty liver disease, 133, 178;
glucose production, storage, and
release, 14, 39, 41, 42, 47, 128, 161;
insulin resistance, 20, 46–47, 53;
insulin sensitivity, 14, 41, 154, 155
lower back, injuries and pain, 73–74,
96–97
lungs: cancer, 232, 247–48, 250;
function, 62, 91, 219; respiratory
diseases, 29, 50, 89, 90, 234, 255

macronutrients, 128–29, 130
magnesium, 55, 110, 140, 234
magnetic resonance imaging (MRI), 94
maltose, 14, 133
mammograms, 6, 249

INDEX • 353

marijuana, 145, 193

meals: bathroom use after, 235; blood glucose levels after, 14, 22–23, 32, 54, 130, 131–32, 156, 239, 254; forgetting to eat, 205; insulin release after, 25; insulin therapy and, 162–63, 164, 166, 168

medical checkups, 6, 87–89

Medicare, 4, 31

medications: accumulation in body fat, 149, 180; adverse health effects/side effects, 4, 18, 29, 30–32, 51, 95–96, 146, 190–91, 200, 224, 258, 341; for bone health, 269; contraindicated in older individuals, 341; as contraindication to alcohol, 136; dosages, 180, 190–91, 236; interactions, 11, 31, 142–43, 145, 151, 224, 279, 342; inventory, 144, 145, 266, 282; management of, 144–52, 205, 266; for mental health issues, 32; metabolism, 149; multiple (polypharmacy), 6, 144, 146, 224, 236, 264–65; obstacles to taking, 16, 29; overmedication, 6; physical activity/exercise and, 168–72. *See also* glucose-lowering medications; prescription medications

meglitinides, 155, 156, 165

melatonin, 219–20, 222, 224

memories, 199, 201, 218, 219

memory, 59; exercises, 105, 210–13; maintenance, 208–14, 283; short- and long-term, 198, 210

memory loss, 11, 29, 150, 195–96, 198–201, 205, 264, 278; long-term, 198; medical or psychological causes, 198–99, 200–201, 243; mild cognitive impairment, 198–99, 201–3; normal levels, 198–200; as obstacle to diabetes management, 203; prevention, 121, 210–13, 265, 266; reversible causes, 198–201, 202–3, 228; short-term, 198

menopause and postmenopause, 52, 91, 138, 173, 267, 269–70

mental health, 108, 207–14, 216, 219, 230; relation to cognitive ability, 194–95

mental stress, 8; adverse health effects, 8, 42, 44, 48–49, 52–53, 109, 134, 198–99, 200, 219, 220; alcohol consumption and, 134–35; diabetes-related ("diabetes distress"), 15, 16, 27, 55, 225–28; stress management strategies, 44, 53, 59, 107, 184, 208, 215, 216, 219, 224–29, 233

metabolic diseases, 21, 42, 53, 54, 108–9, 200

metabolic rate, 61

metabolism, 136, 179–80, 187, 219

metformin, 25, 154, 169; combination therapy, 158; "off-label" use, 154; side effects, 4, 139, 146, 199

metoclopramide, 146

micronutrients, 136

minerals, dietary, 21, 52, 54, 55, 75, 110, 141, 148, 182

mobility impairments, 29, 56, 100, 178, 260, 264, 265, 274, 276

monitoring, of blood glucose levels, 17, 23, 29, 33–37, 205, 238; continuous and intermittent (CGM) systems, 35–36, 164, 223–24; finger-stick monitors, 17, 22, 33–34

monosaccharides, 13–14

Morley, John, 199; *The Science of Staying Young,* 208–9

mortality causes: chronic diseases, 50; in older adults, 7

Munshi, Medha, 1, 2–3

muscle(s): aches/pain/soreness, 51, 73–74, 80, 81, 89, 91–92, 99, 169, 224; body fat storage in, 46, 188; cellular repair, 229–30; cramps, 140, 169; exercise-related damage, 73, 92; fiber types, 63–65, 67; glycogen

354 • INDEX

muscle(s) (*cont.*)
  metabolism and storage in, 39–40,
  64, 65, 81, 161, 162, 165; insulin
  resistance, 20, 46; insulin sensitivity,
  154; oral diabetes medication action
  in, 153; rebuilding (hypertrophy), 92,
  229; statins-related damage, 169
muscle mass: blood glucose storage in,
  31–32; effect of physical activity on,
  6, 58, 61, 62, 74, 172–73, 179, 229,
  233; loss of, 9–10, 74, 91, 172, 182,
  229, 264, 282; loss prevention and
  reversal, 11, 16, 100, 192–93, 266;
  relation to BMI, 186; role in insulin
  resistance management, 47; sarcopenia (age-related muscle wasting),
  9–10, 59, 62, 72, 74, 173, 174, 178,
  179, 190, 191–92, 261, 264–65
muscle-strengthening training. *See*
  resistance training

naproxen sodium, 95, 278
National Institutes of Health, 186
nausea and vomiting, 139, 146, 159,
  191, 246, 252, 253, 341
nerves/nervous system, 3, 22, 43,
  548–49, 1, 91, 101–2, 140; autonomic (central), 121; parasympathetic, 217; sympathetic, 48–49
neuropathy, 112, 137, 139–40;
  autonomic, 69, 82, 121; diabetic, 4,
  88, 142; peripheral, 59, 121
neurotransmitters, 196–97, 199, 206
nonsteroidal anti-inflammatory drugs
  (NSAIDs), 277–78
norepinephrine, 206
nutritional deficiencies, 110, 136–43,
  182, 264–65, 282
nutritional supplements, 55, 141–43,
  144, 145, 148, 282

obesity and overweight, 19–20, 50,
  108–9, 174–75, 177, 181, 185–86,

219, 265; adverse health effects, 50,
  52, 114, 130, 186, 250, 251, 274–75;
  android or gynoid, 187–88
older adults, definition, 4–5
omega-3 and omega-6 fats, 111,
  122–25, 143, 234
oral cancer, 250
oral glucose tolerance test (OGTT),
  22–23, 24, 25, 41
organ damage/failure, 9, 26, 51
orthotics, 71, 277
osteoarthritis, 50, 60, 77, 88, 89, 90,
  171, 234, 274–80, 283
osteopenia, 138, 266, 268
osteoporosis, 231, 236, 266–69,
  272–273, 278–79; prevention or
  reversal, 138, 235, 236, 268–71
over-the-counter medications, 144, 148,
  151, 152, 224, 282
oxidants, 53, 54, 119
oxidative stress, 23, 52, 53, 55, 120, 140,
  203–4, 239
Ozempic, 155, 158, 159

pain: cancer-related, 252; chronic,
  264–65, 266; medications, 22, 71,
  92–93, 171, 277–79
pancreas, 25, 31, 46, 153, 187; cancer,
  248, 250, 255; insulin release from,
  129–30, 152–53, 157; pancreatitis,
  18. *See also* beta cells
pap smears, 249
Parkinson's disease, 146, 197, 200–201,
  206, 342
pelvic floor (Kegel) exercises, 104
peptides, 50–51
periodontal (gum) disease, 231, 235,
  254–57, 283
peripheral artery disease, 242, 243
pesticides, 180, 284, 248
phosphorus, 138, 272
physical activity/exercise, 6, 57–60,
  89, 105–6, 107, 233, 234, 259, 282;

blood glucose level effects, 14, 31–32, 33, 157; for bone health, 269; for cancer prevention, 58, 61, 234, 249, 250; during cancer treatment, 253; for cardiovascular health, 88, 234, 239, 245; cognitive ability benefits, 200, 201, 213–14; with common health problems, 90; cross-training, 56, 97–98; for diabetes management, 11; effect on insulin resistance, 22, 43, 44, 45–46, 47, 54, 160, 183; excessive, 95; for falls prevention, 261–62; for frailty prevention, 266; glucose release in, 14; for inflammation management, 49, 53, 54; for insulin production, 21; insulin therapy and, 70, 102–3, 154, 162, 164–68; for joint and bone health, 58, 60, 61, 62, 67, 69, 71, 75, 234, 235, 269, 276–77; longevity effect, 57, 58; medication use and, 168–72; mental health benefits, 59, 207–8; in mobility-impaired individuals, 56, 66; for muscle mass maintenance, 174, 233; obstacles to, 16, 67, 72, 73, 87; precautions and considerations, 60, 63, 68, 72, 73, 80, 86, 87–97; recommended types for older adults, 65–67, 99–100; rest and recuperation time, 89, 97, 103, 215, 216, 229–30; role in hyperglycemia management, 31–32, 33; for stress management, 226, 228–29; warm-up and cool-down exercises, 71, 86, 91, 95, 96, 101, 102, 103; for weight loss and maintenance, 172, 181–83, 185, 193, 233. *See also* injuries, physical activity/exercise-related

physical inactivity: adverse health effects, 59, 204, 229–30, 267–68; aging-related, 172–73; transitioning to physical activity, 60, 63, 87–89, 99, 105–6

physical therapy, 94–95

phytonutrients, 112, 118–19, 233, 271

pineal gland, 219–20

plantar fasciitis, 93

pollutant exposure, 21

posture, 56, 64, 66; exercises, 74, 84–85, 96, 106

potassium, dietary, 141, 234, 245

prebiotics, 112, 113, 117, 118, 183, 191

prediabetes, 18, 20, 21–25, 41, 43, 87, 176, 219; management, 8, 9–10, 12, 22, 25, 45, 151, 153, 154; reversibility, 22, 38–39, 44, 61; as type 2 diabetes precursor, 20, 21, 181, 266

pregnancy, 35

premature death, 2, 7, 114, 230, 231–32, 268

prescription medications, 145, 146; adverse reactions and side effects risk, 110, 148–51, 180; dosage, 144, 145, 149, 151, 180; generic, 151–52; implications for physical activity, 168–71; interactions, 143, 148, 152; multiple use (polypharmacy), 144, 146, 147–48; safety measures, 146–47, 151–52

preventive approach, to health problems, 6, 231–38; for diabetes, 38–55, 233, 281; screenings/early detection, 6, 185, 233, 234, 236, 237–38, 249, 251

probiotics, 112, 113, 117, 183, 191

proprioception exercises, 83–84

prostate: cancer, 58, 118–19, 247–48, 249–50; benign prostatic hyperplasia, 250–51

protein energy malnutrition, 180

proteins, 140; amino acid component, 18, 127–28; conversion to glucose, 14, 134; dietary intake, 53, 55, 111, 127–28, 133, 134, 174, 235, 271, 272; muscle requirements, 127, 174; stress proteins, 92; supplements, 127–28

356 · INDEX

psychotherapy ("talk therapy"), 207, 221

pulse rate, 3, 29, 69

resistance training, 6, 46, 56, 65, 72–85, 83, 91, 96, 100, 102, 106, 172, 174, 192, 208, 233, 261, 262, 277, 282; as balance training, 82–83, 82–85, 100; for bone mass maintenance, 268–69; for frailty prevention, 266; for injury recurrence prevention, 96; precautions and considerations, 71–72, 79–81; types, 75–77, 303–27; types, lower-body, 76, 313–25; types, upper-body, 76, 303–13

R.I.C.E. techniques (for injuries), 93, 94, 95

RNA, 119, 140

running and jogging, 67, 68, 75, 90, 94, 101, 229

salt/sodium, 54, 141, 185, 234, 235, 245, 272

seizures, 197, 202, 342

selenium, 121, 140, 141, 250

self-care, 5, 15–16

serotonin, 196–97, 206; selective serotonin reuptake inhibitors, 207

SGLT-2 inhibitors, 155, 156–57, 158

shin splints, 93–94

shoulder: flexibility exercises, 86, 87; "frozen," 85, 97, 275; injuries, 96, 97, 101–2; replacement, 87

silent ischemia, 246–47

skin cancer, 232, 247–48, 250

sleep, 215–30; adequate (recommended amount), 48, 97, 224, 233; health benefits, 97, 215–17, 230, 262, 283; non-REM and REM stages, 217–18, 220, 224

sleep disorders/inadequate sleep, 52–53, 60, 198–99, 206, 219, 220, 223–24; adverse health effects, 184, 198–99, 219, 225; insomnia, 51, 141, 220, 221–22; management, 48, 60, 61, 141, 215, 216, 220–24, 228, 283; narcolepsy, 220; REM sleep behavior disorder, 220; restless legs syndrome, 220; sleep apnea, 48, 178, 220, 222–23, 224, 231

smell, sense of, 189, 212, 264

smoking, 6, 52, 88–89, 136, 169, 204, 249, 250, 256, 267–68; cessation, 223, 232, 233, 234, 239, 240, 256

social interactions, 6, 48–49, 205, 213, 258, 259, 264

speech impairments, 247

spine: bone density, 139; degenerative changes/arthritis, 96–97, 276; fractures, 267; stenosis, 171

spirituality and religion, 207, 208–10, 253

statins, 32, 168–69, 239, 241

Stewart, Robert J., 214

strength, aging-related decrease, 90–91

strength training. See resistance training

stress incontinence, 104

stress. See mental stress

stroke, 16, 50, 200–201, 206, 239–40; hemorrhagic, 243; ischemic, 243, 247; risk factors and risk reduction, 22, 118–19, 140, 168–69, 180, 233–34, 239, 243–44, 245; tPA treatment, 243, 247; transient ischemic attacks (TIAs), 244; warning signs (symptoms), 247

sucrose, 14, 133

sugar, 13–14, 54, 132–33, 139, 183, 256; glycemic index, 130, 132

sulfonylureas, 29, 31, 44, 152–53, 155, 156, 157, 158, 165

sunlight exposure, 71, 119, 137–38, 163, 221, 234, 270

suprachiasmatic nucleus, 224

sweating, 29, 185, 246

swimming, 62, 67, 68, 69, 75, 98, 101–2, 105, 229

INDEX · 357

tea, 112, 119, 125
tendinitis, 85, 95, 97; Achilles, 94
tendons, 77, 169, 274
testosterone, 52, 173, 192, 266, 272
thiazides, 32, 170
thiazolidenediones, 155, 157, 158
thirst, increased, 18–19, 23–24
thyroid disease, 261
toxins, 109, 180, 216–17, 234, 248, 250
trigger finger, 185
triglycerides, 46, 180, 199
tumor necrosis factor, 191–92
type 1 diabetes, 2, 3, 18–19, 20, 21, 24, 26, 38, 44, 107, 196, 243, 267; beta cell dysfunction in, 18, 19, 49; blood glucose levels, 27–28, 30, 33, 35, 70; "double diabetes" diagnosis, 41; glucose-lowering drug use in, 154; insulin resistance in, 20, 21, 39, 41, 43; misdiagnosis with type 2 diabetes, 19; osteoporosis risk in, 267; reversibility, 38; symptoms, 18–19, 24; weight-loss diet for, 182. *See also* insulin therapy
type 2 diabetes (adult onset; non-insulin-dependent), 18, 19–21, 24, 107, 127, 178, 185, 186–87, 242, 243, 248; blood glucose levels, 25, 30, 35, 70, 130, 165, 175, 176, 192, 254; insulin resistance in, 22, 39, 41, 43, 44, 48, 49, 118, 127, 130; insulin sensitivity in, 45; misdiagnosis with type 1 diabetes, 19; onset age, 239; prediabetes as precursor to, 20, 21, 181, 266; prevention, 61, 172; reversibility, 20, 21, 22, 38, 44; risk factors, 20, 176, 185–88, 219, 220, 222–23, 255; symptoms, 18–19, 24

US Centers for Disease Control and Prevention, 225–28, 237, 254, 259–60

US Diabetes Prevention Program, 181–82
US Food and Drug Administration, 55, 148, 161, 176, 193, 253, 280
urination: difficulty in, 222; frequency, 17, 18–19, 23–24, 28, 104, 114, 140, 250–51, 260–61, 262; pelvic floor (Kegel) exercises during, 104
urine: blood glucose in, 17, 18–19, 153, 156–57; blood in, 73, 251, 252

vaccinations, 6, 233, 236–37, 249
vascular disease, 89; peripheral, 90, 242, 243
vasodilators, 170
Vinik, Aaron I., 220
vision impairment/eye disorders, 16, 23–24, 28, 88–89, 139, 200, 260–61, 262, 264–65, 266; cataracts, 121, 261, 278–79; risk factors, 26, 29, 32, 43, 140, 243, 247, 252
vitamins, 4, 21, 52, 54, 55, 108, 109, 141, 148, 152, 182; B_1 (thiamine), 139–40; B_2 (riboflavin), 139; B_3 (niacin), 139; B_5 (pantothenic acid), 139; B_6 (pyroxidines), 139; B_9 (folate), 139, 199, 250; B_{12}, 139, 199, 200; B complex, 138–40; C, 121; D, 55, 110, 137–38, 269, 270; D_3, 270; E, 55, 121, 140, 250; K, 108

walkers, 6, 56, 262, 263
walking, 56, 58, 62, 65, 67, 68, 69, 75, 98, 99, 100, 110–11, 242, 246, 263, 264, 277
weight-bearing activities, 75, 91, 98, 174, 268–69
wheelchair users, 56, 65, 80, 100

zinc, dietary, 55, 141–42
zonulin, 110